Extreme
Measures

Extreme Measures

[finding a better path
to the end of life]

Jessica Nutik Zitter, MD

AVERY
an imprint of Penguin Random House
New York

AVERY

An imprint of Penguin Random House LLC
375 Hudson Street
New York, New York 10014

Most Avery books are available at special quantity discounts for bulk purchase
for sales promotions, premiums, fund-raising, and educational needs.
Special books or book excerpts also can be created to fit specific needs.
For details, write SpecialMarkets@penguinrandomhouse.com.

Library of Congress Cataloging-in-Publication Data

Names: Zitter, Jessica Nutik.
Title: Extreme measures : finding a better path to the end of life / by
   Jessica Nutik Zitter, MD, MPH.
Description: New York : Avery, 2017. | Includes index.
Identifiers: LCCN 2016056303 | ISBN 9781101982556 (print)
Subjects: LCSH: Terminal care. | Terminally ill—Care. | BISAC: MEDICAL /
   Terminal Care. | MEDICAL / Ethics. | MEDICAL / Critical Care.
Classification: LCC R726.8.Z58 2017 | DDC 616.02/9—dc23
LC record available at https://lccn.loc.gov/2016056303

Printed in the United States of America
10 9 8 7 6 5 4 3 2 1

BOOK DESIGN BY TANYA MAIBORODA

Brief portions of this book have appeared in *The New York Times, Huffington Post,*
and *Pacific Standard.* Versions here have had redundant portions cut.

TO MY FAMILY:
Mark
and my beloved children,
Solomon, Tessa, and Sasha

In the sufferer let me see only the human being.
MOSES MAIMONIDES

The good physician takes care of the patient's disease,
the great physician takes care of the patient.
WILLIAM OSLER

In order to protect the privacy of my patients and others, identifying details of certain individuals portrayed in the case studies of this book have been changed. These may include, but are not limited to, names, places, dates, family relations, medical details, and locations of care.

Contents

Prefatory Note   *xiii*

[chapter one]   Alone in the Trenches   *1*

[chapter two]   The End-of-Life Conveyor Belt   *19*

[chapter three]   Abandoned in a Sea of Options   *64*

[chapter four]   The Illusion Collusion   *103*

[chapter five]   Where We Come From   *147*

[chapter six]   Who We Are   *182*

[chapter seven]   The Personal Toll   *208*

[chapter eight]   Sharing the Journey   *233*

Epilogue   *279*

[appendix one]   A Way Forward   *289*

[appendix two]   Avoiding Unnecessary Suffering   *298*

Resources   *309*

Notes   *312*

Acknowledgments   *325*

Index   *328*

Prefatory Note

I AM AN ACCIDENTAL EVANGELIST. I didn't set out to change the culture of medicine, my chosen and beloved profession. I just found I had no choice but to try.

Over the course of my career, I have worked in at least twenty hospitals. These include some of the best-known academic medical centers in this country, public hospitals in inner cities, Kaiser Foundation hospitals, and several private facilities. The stories that follow derive from these many different locations. I have seen examples of excellent patient-centered care in each of these and, unfortunately, the contrary as well.

My intention here is neither to cast blame nor to point fingers at any physicians or institutions. In this book, the physician who has been the most insensitive, uttered the most wrong words, and missed the most opportunities to do things right is me.

Rather, this book is about how our collective tendency to

ignore death, doctor and patient alike, fuels a tremendous amount of suffering. And about how we can move forward from this place. I hope that by being as honest as possible about my own shortcomings as well as my changes in thinking along the way, readers will see that we are in the midst of a paradigm shift. None of us has yet "arrived." One of my palliative care colleagues said to me recently, "The only reform that comes is from confession."

And so I've started with myself.

This book is a merging of a few decades of writing and impressions and is not meant to imply that anything is static. My own perspectives have continued to change, as has the culture around me. All for the better. My hope is not to preach but, ultimately, to help us all—patients, families, and health care providers—to construct a more humane approach to helping people as they reach the ends of their lives.

Most of the colleagues I have worked with care deeply. They truly want to deliver care that is more comprehensively oriented toward the patient than they were originally taught to do. But we all work within a system that does not yet readily support us in doing that. And so my message carries their sentiments as well. I am speaking for many people. We are all motivated by the intention to serve in the best way we can.

This is not a textbook. Neither is it a comprehensive methodological approach to changing our culture. It is instead powered by my own interpretations and experiences—the personal reflections of one doctor who is trying to make sense of a very complex and important system that will ultimately affect us all.

chapter one

Alone in the Trenches

July 12, 1992
The second week of my medical internship.

2:45 A.M.

A nurse wakes me up. A patient's Foley, or bladder, catheter has fallen out, and the nurse needs me to put it back in. It is my second week as a medical intern, and her attitude is more like that of a hazing fraternity brother than of a patient advocate. I've been able to lie down for fifteen minutes in the darkened call room on one of the four cots that already smell of other interns' sleep.

10:30 A.M.

I've survived my first night on call but can barely function. I've slept fifteen minutes. The morning hours bear no relief as my pager beeps relentlessly. I make a mental note to answer only every other page and ignore the intervening ones, assuming they'll call back later.

11:45 A.M.

I take the rear stairwell two steps at a time, heading toward my next task on the ninth floor. Mr. A needs to be discharged. That will bring my post-call census down from twenty-one to twenty. I imagine the pen slash I will make as I cross him off my list.

The door slams open above me. Looking up, I see another post-call intern rushing down to attend to something on his list. We grunt at each other. "The only thing we need now is a code," he chortles.

We had all witnessed codes as medical students, standing at the back of the room, small and silent so as not to be ejected by a nurse or, worse, pulled into the fray. Uncapped needles strewn over the bed as a surgical resident tried repeatedly to thread a catheter into a large vein. Chest compressions, violent and exhausting, a relay race of residents and nurses taking turns pumping clotted blood through the patient.

Missing a code was frowned on; every doctor within earshot of the hospital PA system was expected to drop work and show up. Ninety percent of us would quickly be dismissed, but most would remain in the hall chatting, glancing periodically into the room to see whether life or death was winning. It was exhilarating. We believed that by merely following the protocols we'd studied in medical school, we would be able to bring people back from the dead. We'd resuscitate their lifeless bodies with jolts of electricity and chemical cocktails designed to shock the heart out of its complacency. We could reinflate flaccid lungs by thrusting stiff tubes into airways and sending mechanical puffs of air into them, playing them like musical instruments. We'd practiced the various scenarios dozens of times on dummy mannequins, furnished with software showing us the various heart rhythms changing with every treatment we administered. The result was usually the same. The patient's heart rhythm was restored by our efforts. We imagined him waking up from his ordeal, another miracle of modern medicine.

12:30 P.M.

Despite my zeal for my first code, today is not the day. Please, let it wait until tomorrow. I am walking on a high tightrope from which I feel I may tumble with any disturbance. I am on Nine West, standing at the bedside of Mr. A, a homeless man with emphysema. The next unchecked box on my task list reads, "Mr. A, inhaler teaching. Make sure he realizes I have instructed him." If a patient doesn't report on his exit survey that he's been taught how to use his medication, our evaluations suffer. These random surveys keep us on our toes and add to our exhaustive list of boxes to be checked. Mr. A's shaky hands lift the small plastic tool toward his mouth for the fourth time in our unproductive session, as a prematurely ejaculated puff of mist blows off to the right of his face. I am going into my thirtieth hour without sleep and feel like I'm being swallowed by quicksand. I am unable to imagine how I will get this homeless man out of the hospital in the ten minutes I have before my next family meeting. I don't have a ride for him and can't find the social worker to help me get him a taxi voucher.

12:38 P.M.

"Code Blue, eleventh floor." The dreaded words crackle through the speakers, spreading through the corridors like a call to prayer. I feel like fainting. I remember the choreographed response of my residents to code announcements in medical school: Whether buying food in the cafeteria, standing over a patient, or talking on the phone, they lifted their heads toward the operator's voice, cocking them so as not to miss any relevant information. Food trays would be abandoned, phones slammed into their cradles, and patients left speechless in their wake. They were being summoned to save a life.

Now it is my turn. Without explanation, I turn and run out of Mr. A's room. How best to scale the two floors that lie between me and the dying patient? But this concern quickly fades as I am transported toward her by a river of white-clad soldiers, who carry me off into the stairwell. As we sprint up the two flights, our calls ricochet off the narrow walls. What room? Where do we go? Is it your patient? We climb with the urgency of an army on the move and finally explode onto the eleventh floor, the heavy door banging loud against the wall.

I follow the crowd, feeling the eyes of patients and visitors on us as we run through the hall. A tickle of pride is followed by a shot of adrenaline flooding my exhausted body. Nurses wave their arms, ushering us toward the room like ramp agents directing a plane to its berth. I quicken my pace, recalling a scene from some television show in which two medical residents rekindled a dead romance while working side by side to save their patient. That same patient later attended their wedding as an honorary guest. Anything is possible!

And whom will we save? A young pregnant woman with life-threatening asthma? A sixty-year-old man having a terrible heart attack? We will pounce on the patient with the force of super-heroes, I tell myself, each of us with her own expertise, freshly trained, to save the day. There will be a thankful family, who witness the resuscitation because we are too busy to throw them out of the room. They will stand stock-still, wide-eyed and open-mouthed, afraid to move lest they distract us from our mission. They will write accolades about us to the chiefs of our residencies. We will be inducted as lifesavers, our hazing complete and actually, all things considered, not so bad. We will emerge exhausted but magnificent, with our stethoscopes slightly askew.

So it is with astonishment that I lay eyes on the poor soul who is to be the first recipient of my lifesaving efforts. The patient's skin is an ashy gray-yellow with a waxy sheen. The abdomen is visible beneath the soiled sheets, deflated from years of malnourishment and disease. A resident is already doing chest compressions, kneeling on the bed to get better leverage. With each compression, there is a sickening click, which I don't recognize until I hear someone next to me whisper, "His whole chest is breaking." This man is dead. He looks like the cadavers in med school, only less healthy. There is not an ounce of fat or muscle on his skeletal frame. The stench of kidney failure, acrid and vinegary, fills the room. The patient's mouth is slack and loose and keeps slipping out from underneath the mask being used to ventilate him. I am still standing in the doorway, dumbstruck by this Armageddon, when my resident, leaning against the sink with his arms crossed and a cool steady eye on the proceedings, subs me in for chest compressions.

"Jessica, relieve Dara." I approach the body with horror. Dara backs off the bed as I brush past her to resume the compressions. Bone grinds against bone under my palms. One more strong push and I worry I will crush him. I envision my hands breaking into his chest cavity, swamped in blood and tissue. I hold my body rigidly upright to minimize the actual pressure on the patient's chest, while trying to ensure that my compressions still look aggressive. I concentrate on breathing only through my mouth as nausea creeps from my stomach into the back of my throat. I begin to feel dizzy.

"More epi," the resident calls. "And we could try another atropine. How long have we been at this?"

"It's been twenty-two minutes," says the recording nurse.

"Well, let's give it another eight minutes to make it a full half hour," he says, leaning back against the sink.

I don't think I will make it. I have rehearsed for the wrong performance.

The eight minutes crawl by, the patient's chest clicking like the hand of an old clock. Finally, we reach our arbitrary goal of half an hour, a round number that should satisfy the family as well as our colleagues at morning report.

"Let's call it," my resident says. He is still leaning against the sink with his arms crossed.

1:10 P.M.

The surgeons start to clean up the sharps, the nurses disconnect monitors and IVs. I have just assaulted a dead body. I feel a terrible dread about my career choice.

"Did you guys eat yet?" my resident asks. "It's going to be a busy day if it continues like this."

I Always Wanted to Save Lives

There is a photograph of me in diapers listening intently to my bear's leg through my father's black stethoscope. Descending from two generations of surgeons on my father's side, I yearned to join their club. My father, grandfather, and a host of great-uncles were scrappy doctors who prided themselves on their technical skills and calm in the face of death. Their patients honored them with a continuous holiday stream of wine, chocolate, and smoked fish.

But it hadn't always been that way. Mine was a family of recent immigrants escaping the poverty and anti-Semitism of Eastern Europe. They came to Montreal to tend fruit stands, butcher stalls, and other small businesses, working late into the night and struggling to put bread on the table for their families. One of my great-grandfathers was a tailor; the other ran a small millinery store. Although they struggled, they gave everything they had to hoist the next generation up into the light. They would not be satisfied with a modicum of comfort and safety but instead worked relentlessly to enable those of us coming after to become educated and respectable members of our new community.

It took only one generation for that to happen. Of the eight sons born to my father's four grandparents, four became doctors and two dentists. The other two helped their father with his tailoring business.

A professional education was the Holy Grail. "You just need the piece of paper," my maternal grandfather would say in broken English, regarding diplomas. And a medical diploma was the best paper of all. The Jewish comedian Jackie Mason jokes about the expectations Jewish parents placed on their children when he was growing up in Brooklyn. The best ones, he says, were expected to be doctors. Those that couldn't make it were to be lawyers, "and if his mind don't work at all, an accountant." But all good humor stems from the truth. This drive to educate children, preferably as doctors, was, at least in my family, overarching and all-powerful.

And why a doctor? From its inception, Judaism has venerated the practice of medicine. The Torah itself, the central core of its beliefs, glorifies the eradication of disease and the sanctity of life. God states in Exodus 23, "I shall remove illness from your midst." In Deuteronomy 7 we are reassured that "Hashem [God] will remove from you every illness."

And the Talmud, which interprets the Torah's instructions into a code of laws for the Jewish people, formalizes the high value placed on the act of lifesaving. It states, "Whoever saves a life, it is considered as if he saved an entire world." Anyone acting to save a life is permitted to break almost any Jewish law. Even the laws of the holy Sabbath could be put aside in favor of life-saving activities—it is considered "God's work." In fact, it is required that any law conflicting with life or health be broken; "he who asks questions sheds blood," says a tractate of Jewish law. In other words, hesitation of any sort to save a life renders one complicit.

And the doctor was therefore introduced as God's agent for healing. Being a doctor was considered a profession of communal importance similar to that of a rabbi. So it should come as no surprise that over millennia, Jews have gravitated toward this calling in notably high proportions relative to the general population. At least whenever they were permitted. One might trace the history of anti-Semitism by examining the peaks and valleys of our participation in the field of medicine. Jewish physicians were well respected in ancient Greece and Europe, serving many of the highest officials in those lands. But beginning in the fourth century C.E., the church and various governments began to place restrictions on their abilities to matriculate and practice as doctors. Innumerable regulations, papal bulls, and royal ordinances forbade Jewish physicians to treat non-Jews, to study at universities, and to hold any official positions. This form of anti-Semitism existed in various forms and places until modern times. In fact, McGill University, where most of my family members were educated, imposed a 10 percent quota on Jewish students beginning in 1920 that lasted until the 1960s, right around the time my father began his training in neurosurgery.

And it was not about the money. At least not in my family. My grandfather's and great-uncles' practices were filled with working-class and poor patients. There was a sliding scale for payment. My grandfather charged $600 to deliver the child of a wealthy person and $150 for someone in the middle class. The poor didn't pay at all. He was paid in cash, $10 at a time or whatever someone could afford. My uncle remembers the large wad of ten-dollar bills in the top drawer of my grandfather's desk. There were times when my grandfather ripped up invoices for poor people, telling his secretary, "You can't send this!" According to family lore, at his death, he was hundreds of thousands of dollars in arrears. My uncle Arnold, who became a family practitioner in Jamaica, Queens, cared for mostly poor and impoverished patients. He received mostly fivers for his work. For these men, being a doctor was about knowledge culled from the pages of medical books, about skill, and, most important, about being of service to others.

My mother's side of the family was a generation behind. Her parents were both immigrants from Europe, neither with any college or professional education. They worked long hours in their clothing store, saving everything they could for their three daughters' education. And their work paid off. Sandra, the eldest daughter and matchmaker to my parents, graduated from medical school in my father's class. I'll never forget how on the night before starting medical school, in a state of anxious insomnia, I sat in my new, shared apartment and opened a coffee table book belonging to my roommate called *The Family of Woman*. I flipped from page to page, seeing photographs of women of all sorts. I paused on a page with a photograph of a woman pediatrician, gloriously pregnant, using a bright light to look into the throat of a crying two-year-old. She stuck out her own tongue playfully to the child. I smiled at the photo, feeling that this was somehow a good omen. And then I looked closer. The pediatrician on the page was my own auntie Sandra. I began to laugh. I was still nervous about what was in store for me, but I felt solace. This would be a homecoming of sorts.

Although late to the game, my mother, Rhoda, was also

drawn to this vocation. As a practicing biochemist, at the age of forty-eight she was accepted to Case Western Reserve University School of Medicine, in the class two years behind me. I had the honor as an alumna of handing my mother her medical diploma at her graduation.

AS THE FIRST GRANDCHILD ON both sides of this family, I was convinced from my earliest days that I would enter the medical profession. No one pushed me. There were no stipulations. It just felt like my destiny. Except for a short, rebellious dalliance during my senior year of college with the idea of becoming a rabbi, medicine as a career was a no-brainer. I think it was the stories that did it, the ones that celebrated the diagnostic acumen of quick thinkers, the extensive knowledge gleaned from the study of medical texts, and the confidence my forebears inspired in those around them. And the heroism of it all.

There was Uncle Harry, my paternal grandfather's brother, on loan as a surgeon to the British by the Canadian Army during World War II. He served as a lieutenant under General Montgomery, seeing action in Syria, North Africa, and Italy and coming back a captain. During the war, while heading the 866 Field Dressing Station, an "advanced surgical and blood transfusion unit," he learned the art of triage. This protocol, whereby doctors determine how to allocate precious resources using a rapid assessment of the patient, is something we take for granted in today's world: who will benefit from immediate treatment, who can wait for a while, and who will surely die. He brought these skills back with him to the Jewish General Hospital, where he worked first as a general surgeon and then as the director of the emergency room.

Many years later, Uncle Harry saved his own life in an act of profound heroism. As he walked out the doors of the emergency room on his way home one evening, he felt a ripping sensation in his midchest. He knew immediately that his aorta, the central conduit of all blood flow out of the heart, was shearing. A rupturing aortic aneurism is almost universally fatal. He stumbled back in the doors, called for one of his staff physicians, and calmly directed him to summon the thoracic surgery team at once. He was on the operating table within fifteen minutes and found to have a critical aortic tear. His life was saved due to his quick action and diagnostic acumen. Had he made it twenty feet farther out of the hospital before his aortic dissection, he would never have survived. He recovered well and went on to live another decade. But that story will never die.

Another great-uncle, my grandmother's brother Samson, was drafted by the U.S. Marine Corps as an oral surgeon during the Korean campaign. Once there, he was unexpectedly appointed acting commander of a MASH unit serving the 45th Thunderbird Division after the commanding officer died. His life was interrupted for sixteen months as he performed his duties, leaving a wife to fend for herself with two toddlers. But he credits that time with making him a great oral surgeon.

These are just a few of the oft-repeated stories that were part of the soundtrack of my childhood. Looking back, I realize that I had been rehearsing to take my place in the family business from almost the beginning. As a young child, I would pull my father's medical books off the shelf and look at pictures of diseased people, daring myself to keep turning the pages. In elementary school, I marked the days until the times when my father's call schedule intersected with a weekend. On those special occasions, my mother would pack a picnic lunch and we would head over to the Montreal Neurological Institute to meet him. A thermos of macaroni and cheese, the wax paper with sliced cucumbers, and a straw-ready milk carton—I was in heaven. On the rare days when the weather was not too frigid, we headed up to the roof for a picnic. The best moment was when my father, in his scrubs, would join us, cool and calm, even though he had important things to do.

Later still, I gained a reputation as the only girl who didn't flinch when we dissected frogs in biology class. I willed myself not to look away when holding my father's research cats, with their horrifying scars and staple lines, attesting to unknown surgeries on their little brains. I was meant for this profession.

My Grandfather's Hands

Oscar Nutik's office was on the first floor of the house. The entry landing had a short staircase, which went down to the waiting room, and another short staircase going up to the house. The sweet hint of pipe smoke puffed out of the cool leather chairs when you took a seat in the waiting room. Only quiet voices were tolerated near the waiting room, and regular shushing could be heard from all of the female members of my family. Grampa's office was treated as sacred space. And Grampa's work was considered similarly awesome. My father tells of a day when he was in his teens. His father had come up from his clinic for dinner. He stood at the kitchen sink and performed the usual six-minute surgeon's hand wash, his forearms carefully lathered, his nailbrush dripping on the sink ledge. My grandmother rushed around the kitchen, assembling his meal.

After he had completed the ritual, shaking excess water into the sink with a neat flick of his wrists, he looked around for the fresh towel usually placed preemptively on the counter next to him by my grandmother. It wasn't there. This had never happened before. And it never would again. He stood in disbelief with his arms elevated, surgeon style, waiting for assistance. He was hissing quietly, through clenched lips that displayed his fury. "Ann! Where is my towel? My hands are getting chapped!" The hands that fed a family, that saved lives, delivered babies. My grandmother ran around him, clucking accusingly at herself, quickly encasing his arms in a warm, fresh towel.

Hearing this story as a teenager, I knew which side of the towel I wanted to be on. And I'm sure my grandmother wanted the same for me.

My Father's Magic Briefcase

Some girls played with Barbie. I played with my father's doctor bag.

I spent many a rainy afternoon between the ages of four and ten splayed out on the floor with his neurology bag. It was like something from *Get Smart,* an ordinary, hard-sided attaché case that my father carried to and from work. I would lay it gently on the rug in our living room, press the buttons, and listen for the satisfying flick of the spring-loaded brass catches on either side of the handle.

Inside the case lay a plastic organizer, the type you might find in a cutlery drawer, which fit snugly, to the millimeter. Within each of the organizer's compartments sat a mysterious tool with moving parts, each with its own set of special instructions, unwritten, but passed from trainer to trainee, father to daughter. Repeatedly I asked my father for these instructions, and he never tired of demonstrating the accoutrements of his trade, explaining—in increasingly complex terms as I grew older—their various uses for diagnosing the multitude of neurological disorders that might afflict a patient.

There were the colored glasses, which resembled swim goggles except that one lens was red, the other green. A doctor could diagnose subtle dysfunction of the nerves or muscles of the eyes by asking the be-goggled patient to look, first to one side and then to the other, and report which color was seen in each direction. There was a piece of material that looked like a power necktie, with red and white diagonal stripes. My father taught me how to anchor one end in the groove between my thumb and forefinger, and then slowly slide the length of it horizontally for my patient to watch. He demonstrated optokinetic nystagmus, a normal reflex where your eye first moves along with the fabric, then flips back repeatedly to the originating side. That reflex, he explained, is lost with certain lesions of the brain. Today, such lesions can usually be diagnosed by a CT scan or MRI, but in those days such diagnoses required the skills and artistry of a Sherlock Holmes. The ophthalmoscope, too complicated to master given my youthful lack of hand–eye coordination, had a bright light that would narrow or widen as I rotated the wheel. There was a two-point discriminator, resembling a compass used in geometry, for testing sensory levels, and a tuning fork that I used to tune every piece of furniture in our house. And a used Kodak film canister that held a soggy piece of sponge soaked with the scent of eucalyptus, to test the olfactory nerve. And, of course, the reflex hammer, which brought on uproarious laughter until someone got hurt.

This bag of tricks was more than just a toy for me. It earned me a wealth of affirmation from my family. And provided a taste of what it would feel like to actually be a doctor. The positive feedback. The mysterious rituals and promise. The sense that if I could just master these tools, I would have something to offer.

A Trip to the Emergency Room

As my seven-year-old body careened down the steep driveway, racing toward the quickly approaching stone wall, I realized my lapse in judgment. But it was too late. My scalp was lacerated, and blood streamed into my eyes. My father was quickly summoned. Family lore tells of my abrupt change in attitude when I realized my luck. My sobbing dried up almost instantly as I understood that I would be taken to the hospital. And with my father no less. And Uncle Harry, my grandfather's brother, a surgeon and the director of the ER at the Jewish General Hospital, would make a special trip to see me.

"Can we see the cats?" My father's research cats made great playmates, seeking affection and companionship even with their zippers of stitches. No, I was told. We had to rush and see Uncle Harry in the emergency room. He would stop the bleeding on my head. We didn't have time to see the kitties.

It didn't matter. I was going to the hospital! I eagerly jumped into the car holding bloody towels to my head. When we arrived, an entourage of nurses surrounded me. I was royalty, a Nutik, whose father, grandfather, uncle, and great-uncle were institutions within an institution. The nurses jumped at their curt commands.

Uncle Harry moved around the room quietly, drawing lido-caine into glass syringes. He didn't talk to me or to my father. This was serious business, and I realized that there was no socializing to be done. Crying was not an option. I waited quietly, my little heart pounding, as Uncle Harry tilted the chair back and removed the crusty towel. "She's going to need at least seven." Stitches, I realized. I'd had a friend who had received stitches recently. She'd been terrified. She'd cried and screamed. In the end, she'd been bribed with candy and presents. But I wouldn't be *that* girl. Despite my terror, I realized my opportunity. I would be brave. I would make them proud. I would follow those who had gone before me and show them what I was made of. My father lounged against the countertop across the room. "Is it going to be okay?" I asked him quaveringly. "Sure," he said with a chuckle, "it's going to be fine." Indeed, except for a tiny scar beautifully tucked under my hairline, it was fine.

But looking back so many years later, the terror of being on that side of the needle is still palpable. I remember the loneliness as I sat in the cold chair, under the bright lights. I remember bracing for pain, the needle glinting in my uncle's gloved hand. I remember the silence, the expectation that I would play my part without complaining, without questioning. I remember the powerlessness and the distance. In those moments, I learned that good doctors don't need to talk to you. They just need to do their job. And you need to trust them. And if that contract is followed, things will turn out for the best. If you cry or ask questions, you just delay the inevitable and gum up the works.

MOST OF MY ROLE MODELS were surgeons, strong and silent. Before medical school, I had assumed I too would be a surgeon. It felt like my destiny: the surgical knots I had practiced with my father, my family's reverence of the profession, and the many who had come before me.

But it became clear to me during my third-year surgical clerkship that I did not want to be a surgeon. The culture felt too aggressive, even bullying, and the hierarchy oppressive. And so after medical school, I entered training in internal medicine. But as I approached the end of my residency, I realized that I was still drawn toward the more invasive fields. And so I chose to pursue fellowship training in pulmonary and critical care medicine, the most heroic and invasive of the medical subspecialties. Like surgery, it valued swiftness, certainty, and the saving of lives. I liked its focus on the sickest patients, trying to bring them back to safety using miracle technologies and Hail Mary passes. I saw it as the ultimate hero's specialty.

It would even enable me to save my grandmother's life.

DOCTORS FOUND A LARGE MASS in my maternal grandmother's abdomen. It was curable, they said, and with surgery she should do well. As a third-year medical resident, I was elected by the family to fly to Montreal, where I would keep a medical "eye on things." The surgery went smoothly—we all breathed a sigh of relief. The next day, my aunt and I went to the hospital for what we expected would be a quick good-bye on our way to the airport. But something was wrong.

My grandmother couldn't talk and mumbled incoherently. It was Thanksgiving Day and there was only a skeleton staff present. Her urine bag was empty and the blood pressure cuff in the room didn't register a pressure. My worst fears were confirmed. She was in septic shock—dying.

None of the surgical residents was answering his pager, so I commandeered the floor nurse. My grandmother needed fluid, I told her, a lot of fluid, or she would surely die. I managed to convince her, and the nurse began a rapid infusion of fluids. I then paged the attending physician myself, explaining the urgent situation. My grandmother was prepped and draped in the operating room within thirty minutes. A four-hour surgery ensued.

She went on to live another ten years, saw the birth of two grandchildren, and died with her children at her side.

Saving my grandmother's life was a defining moment. My lifesaving skills had been put to the best use imaginable. I had clearly chosen the right path. In my mid-twenties, I was in training at a prestigious internal medicine residency in Boston. Most of my friends from college were still finding their ways professionally, sampling jobs that might or might not launch them onto a career path. Being able to say, "I'm a medical resident at the Brigham" was calming. The physical exhaustion, the stress of being called on in morning report, the mental overload of handling multiple sick patients, these were nothing compared to the anxiety I would have felt had I been another college graduate searching for a professional identity. I tied up many loose ends in my young life by choosing medicine. I would always be able to support myself. I would never have to take chances if I didn't want to. I would be consumed by a demanding training for years to come. I would be seen as a success—by others and by myself. I felt for my nonmedical friends in times when they reached dead ends and needed to retrace steps and launch into new directions. They envied my scrubs, my beeper importantly peeking out of a slightly untucked shirt, my clean elevator pitch of what I did for a living. I would have too, if I were they.

That was my thinking until the afternoon I performed chest compressions on a dead patient.

chapter two

The End-of-Life Conveyor Belt

T HE PATIENT HAD BEEN on the regular hospital ward for weeks. The latest round of chemotherapy for her metastatic breast cancer had severely damaged her kidneys, causing a host of serious problems which had now turned critical. She was transferred from the floor to room 5 in the intensive care unit (ICU) for more aggressive treatment. As her bed whizzed into the unit, propelled by the ward attending, he looked up at me. "She needs dialysis. I called renal, and they'll do it as soon as you get the dialysis catheter in."

It was 2003 and I was a new attending at University Hospital in Newark, New Jersey. *Let's get to it,* I thought. I sat down with our team's medical student to scan the patient's chart. Not only were the patient's kidneys failing but her liver was shutting down as well. The acid level in her blood was dangerously high. And her blood pressure had plummeted dangerously low. *There is probably no turning this around,* I thought. But we might as well give it a try.

First step, I told my student, is to check the patient's blood clotting parameters. "We don't want to trigger a bleed on top of everything else," I said. Next, we needed to get consent from the husband, who was standing nervously at her bedside. The student followed me into the room, and I introduced myself to the husband. Both of his hands were clenched tightly around the guardrail of the bed. "Sir, your wife's kidneys have stopped working," I said, "so we're going to need to do dialysis to clean her blood. The first step is placing a catheter into this vein in her neck." I pointed to my own internal jugular vein under my jaw.

He nodded, his face white. "Do you need me to leave now?"

"Not yet," I said, and went on to list the risks of the procedure, checking them off on my fingers one by one. Pneumothorax, bleeding, infection of the site. I described each of these and, in the same breath, how we would manage it. He looked terrified, but he nodded and signed the form. We told him we would bring him back from the waiting room once the line was placed.

The student and I gathered the various accoutrements for the procedure from different carts around the ICU. I instructed him on the importance of placing the waterproof "chux" sheet underneath the impending surgical site to catch any blood or fluid that might result from the procedure. "You really want to keep the nurses on your side," I said, "and a messy sheet means the whole bed needs to be changed." Then I cleared off the rolling bedside table and placed the catheter kit on top. "This is the Quinton catheter," I said. I pulled off the top layer of the kit and then, after donning sterile gloves, proceeded to unfold the blue paper wrapping so the inner tray sat like a treasure chest in the middle of the sea. "You're going to want to follow the set of steps that I teach you in sequence each time," I said. I proceeded to set up the kit, filling its syringes with lidocaine and saline and flushing the catheter to ensure its ports were functioning. Then I proceeded to clean the surgical site by turning the patient's head to the left in order to better access the large neck vein below her right jaw. I swabbed the area with widening circles of Betadine three times. Then it was time to enclose myself within the sterile field. This is a procedure whereby the operator encloses herself in a sterile gown and gloves in order to prevent even the slightest chance of bacteria coming into contact with the surgical site. I pulled off the Betadine-stained gloves with a quick snap. Gathering my hair in a bun, I slipped on a bouffant cap, then tied a mask over my mouth. Next I opened the package containing a sterile gown, touching only the inner side of it so as to keep the outside sterile, and stood in the center of the room to shake it open. I wriggled into it. The nurse moved behind me and quickly fastened the ties at the back of the gown. I pushed my hands through to don the sterile gloves that lay waiting on sterile paper in front of me. The nurse handed me one end of a sterile half-size surgical drape. Being careful that my gloves did not touch her hand, I moved away from her, spreading the drape over the patient. Now it was time to take my place at the head of the patient's bed. The ICU nurse pushed the bedside table, covered in its own drape, right up next to the bed so that it stood beside the patient's right arm, another Lego piece of blue sterility snapped into place. I asked the nurse to tilt the head of the bed down below the foot into a position called Trendelenburg. This increases the pooling of blood in the neck in order to facilitate access to the vein.

And then I saw Pat. She was leaning against the doorjamb and she looked furious. *Oh crap*, I thought to myself. *Here we go again.*

Five foot ten inches tall with a strawberry blond bob, Pat loomed at the door in her white coat. The woman had nothing if not presence.

Pat Murphy was an advanced practice registered nurse (APRN) who now ran the recently formed Family Support Team in our ICU. I didn't know much about it, except that suddenly there were people with clipboards looking over our shoulders and talking to our patients. And somehow I found myself feeling judged.

The team's message to us was that our patients needed more information and support than we doctors were giving them. Unlike most nurses I had worked with, Pat called it as she saw it, within earshot or not, and without regard for the hierarchical structure of ICU culture, where doctors' words were gospel. She and her team of tough New Jersey women entered rooms without our permission, talked to our patients without asking, and wrote recommendations on the chart like a regular medical consult team.

Although I'm embarrassed to say it now, in those early days I mostly viewed the Family Support Team as superfluous at best and problematic at worst. I believed I was doing just fine communicating with my patients. I had done advanced fellowship training in the management of failing organs so, in all fairness, how could Pat provide options better than mine?

The whole idea of bringing someone else into the covenantal relationship between a doctor and her patient felt destabilizing to me. Suddenly someone else was in the room, upsetting the equilibrium, encouraging new types of questions we didn't have answers to, laying out new options that were not part of the well-worn protocols we doctors had mastered. And where would Pat be, I'd fret, while I was trying to clean up the mess she had made? She'd be on to the next patient, rabble-rousing and leaving me to deal with the fallout.

And what if, as a result of Pat's involvement, the patient decided he didn't want the treatments I was offering? What would I do for that patient whose lungs were failing if not to attach him to a breathing machine? Just let him die? Where? Would I send him out from the ICU to the hospital ward? And what would my colleagues think of me for giving up on prolonging life at all costs? Would the family sue me? Would I need to require the patient to sign legal forms saying he had elected not to pursue treatments I felt were warranted? I worried that if patients listened to Pat, they would be left in a no-man's land, with no tether to the world they had sought out for help.

And now Pat stood in the doorway, tapping her foot. On her face was a mixture of horror and resignation. I refocused my attention on the patient. She was moaning but still, her face covered under the thick paper drapes. As I prepared to insert a large needle into her neck, Pat lifted an imaginary phone to her ear. "Nine-one-one, get me the police," she said, glaring at me. "They're torturing a patient in the ICU at University Hospital."

I paused, stunned. And suddenly I realized that she was absolutely right. I stood motionless, needle hovering.

Over my years in training I had had many moments of profound disillusionment. Moments when I had doubted that my efforts were helping my patients—worried, in fact, that I was actually hurting them. But I was able to brush them away by running off to my next urgent assignment.

Yet this encounter hit me like a punch in the gut. Instead of resentment, I felt shame. The patient under the hot drapes; was I really helping her? Of course not. I knew, as did everyone else involved in her care, that she had only days left of life. And every second under the hot drapes was another second separated from her anxious husband in the waiting room, who wanted nothing more than to be by her side.

But I couldn't see a way out of the situation. It had already gone too far. My drive—no, my compulsion—to continue to "treat" her was so deeply ingrained that I could not yet imagine another role for myself. And what would I say to her husband, the nurses, and the medical student at my side, all waiting expectantly for me to complete the ritual we had all subscribed to? The sterile field had been painstakingly prepared, and now I stood trapped in it. I stared at the moaning lump of patient, supine beneath the blue drapes, and mentally ran through the various options. I could leave the sterile field in place, remove my gown and gloves, and go find the husband in the waiting room. What would I tell him? That my recommendation that we insert this catheter had been based solely on assessing the turgor pressure of her vascular system, not on the likelihood of actually making her better? Would I admit that she was actually dying and that all of the things we were doing were essentially distractions from this reality? Confess that in my zeal to *do something*, I had led him to a treatment that would do nothing more than hurt his wife in her final hours? And what about the nurse and medical student waiting in the room for me to complete the procedure? How long should I tell them to wait? How long before the sterility of the field expired and we would need to redo the entire proceedings? On top of everything, the dialysis nurse was now outside the room with her machine, waiting to connect it to the catheter in the patient's neck. She had pushed this patient to the top of the schedule, at our request. What would I tell her? All of these adjustments risked making me appear wimpy and discombobulated, I felt. I believed that an ICU doctor must never show second thoughts or self-doubt. Never let them see you sweat. But now I felt my face covered by a thin layer of mist.

I steeled myself. I'd put my patient on this path, and it felt

EXTREME MEASURES

beyond my abilities at this point to change direction. I had to move, and the only way I could see was forward. I took in a deep breath, pulled the skin taut beneath the patient's jaw, and inserted the needle.

Pat walked out, shaking her head. Her words hung in the air like a judge and jury.

That catheter didn't prolong the patient's life. But it changed mine.

THE SEEDS OF THE MODERN ICU were sown in the late 1930s and 1940s. The polio epidemic was felling young bodies left and right, as such scourges had done over the course of human history. But this time there was the Drinker respirator, better known as the iron lung. Developed in 1928 by an industrial hygienist at the Harvard School of Public Health, it was powered by a simple engine and air pumps from two vacuum cleaners, which created a rhythmic vacuum around the patient's torso to ease inhalation. They cost as much as the average home in 1930, but in actuality, they were priceless: In the 1940s and 1950s, later models of these metal boxes kept many thousands of people alive while their bodies fought the polio virus. Thus began our love affair with medical technology. As Larry Alexander wrote in his book, *The Iron Cradle: My Fight against Polio,*

> The metal respirator assumed an almost animate personality and became a symbol of protection and security. . . . We were incomplete embryos in a metal womb.

The machines required space and skilled personnel to do their work, leading to the birth of the modern ICU and, with it, the field of pulmonary and critical care medicine. Polio victims in iron lungs lined the ICUs of hospitals around the United States, each spending on average a week before regaining enough strength to breathe unassisted. Many would then go on to live full, healthy lives.

In the mid-twentieth century, mobile army surgical hospitals, or MASH units, were appearing on the battlefields of World War II and Korea. These temporary hospitals were sometimes erected as close as ten miles from the fighting. Soldiers dying of hemorrhage or infection were rushed to these units to receive lifesaving blood, plasma, and fluids. Doctors began to perfect the art of blood pressure monitoring and resuscitation. Many young lives were saved that in previous generations would have been lost. Medical technology was accomplishing the unimaginable.

If a little is good, a lot must be better. Soon, ICUs were everywhere. By the end of the 1960s most hospitals had at least one. And then came a veritable alphabet soup of options for special circumstances: The surgical ICU (SICU), the pediatric ICU (PICU), the neonatal ICU (NICU), the postanesthesia ICU (PACU), the cardiac ICU (CICU), and on and on. There is even a digestive diseases ICU (DDICU) at the Medical University of South Carolina.

By 2014, there were more than 77,000 ICU beds for just 5,600 hospitals in the United States. ICUs were spawning. They continue to proliferate at an astounding rate, growing by 7 percent between 2000 and 2005. Our country houses many more ICU beds per capita than other comparable nations. The ICU became revered as medicine's silver bullet. You go in almost dead, you come out alive.

But there was a catch. Our infatuation with the ICU and its machines caused us to use them indiscriminately. If they could help a young child or a soldier, why not try them on everyone who is dying? And so we did. In the name of hope, heroism, and the American way.

The first two years of medical school were as expected for an earnest and humanistically inclined medical student. We spent a lot of time in lectures, cramming knowledge about physiology into the crevices of our brains. But as we collected our notes and flashcards and took our tests, we were impatient to be introduced to *the patient,* the reason most of us went to medical school in the first place.

We would have to wait until the second semester of the first year. By then, we would have been introduced to the tools of our trade—the stethoscopes, otoscopes, and ophthalmoscopes—that might help us diagnose whatever was ailing our patient. As I learned to handle the devices, fumbling at first but soon maneuvering them as if they were extensions of my own arm, the glee of those childhood afternoons with my father's attaché case transformed into a different kind of joy. I was becoming a doctor.

In the beginning, we practiced on each other. That first barrier, where one would lay hands on another, was particularly bizarre. Just out of college, few of us had ever touched another human being in this way—it wasn't about love, or sex, or the neediness of a child, but something else. We needed to cultivate our "doctor hands," as I thought of it, through which we would be able to touch another person without sensuality, while disguising any discomfort or aversion we might feel. On the first day of our physical exam block, as we sat in the lecture hall grasping our stethoscopes, our professor called for a volunteer. A male, who would be willing to take his shirt off and be examined by us all. There was a long and uncomfortable silence. Eventually Louis, an attractive student whom I hardly knew, stepped awkwardly up to the stage. I barely breathed as I held my stethoscope to his chest. Today, I am able to put on my doctor hands to examine any part of any person's body in the blink of an eye, no matter whether it be a patient, a friend, or a family member. But this was a skill that required repeated practice over the first few years of my medical training.

Doctor hands were, in a sense, just another tool. Learning our role in the doctor–patient relationship, however, was far more complex. Most of us had come to medical school for humanistic reasons. We wanted to help. But, we were cautioned, it was critical to learn how to situate our empathy within professional boundaries. You couldn't spend all of your time with one patient when there were many others who needed you. We were instructed on how to interview patients in ways that brought them into the conversation with us. One of the instructors was famous for her backstage hiss of "open-ended questions, open-ended questions." Cameras would capture us on tape, and we would then watch ourselves as we bumbled through our interview, wrinkling our noses if we misspoke or didn't pick up on a cue from our "patient." By the end of my second year, I felt like I was getting the hang of it.

But things changed abruptly when I began my third-year clerkships, a dizzying sequence of monthlong embeddings with ward teams in different disciplines: internal medicine, surgery, OB-GYN, and others. No longer were my "patients" paid actors and volunteers following predictable scripts, whose assigned diseases usually got better. No longer was I in the shelter of a classroom, solving cases on paper, overseen by physicians who gravitated toward the sensitive mentoring of students and trainees. Rather, I was unceremoniously dumped onto the wards with little guidance or support, faced with real patients, real diseases, and often profound suffering.

There I trailed behind a medical team composed of an attending doctor who was generally present only for rounds, a harried resident responsible for innumerable details, and a couple of sleep-deprived and overwhelmed interns. I wore the short white coat of a student, which advertised that I had almost nothing to offer. I felt like an idiot. Every note I wrote, interview I conducted, or differential diagnosis I conjured felt wrong, off base, naive. I couldn't help but notice the team's polite disinterest in my detailed presentation of a patient's social history, the only part of the case I could present with any confidence.

Until then, I had had no idea of the full scope of human suffering. I was suddenly witness to misery, death, and raw emotion. None of my close family members had ever been hospitalized and I had attended only one funeral, that of my aged grandfather. How could I presume to help these patients and grieving families? I was Student Doctor Nutik, with no real skills or experience. And so I generally stood back from the patients and families, whose needs seemed too vast for me to fill in any way.

Worse, I felt completely isolated. I had no one to talk to about my own shock and sadness. My mentors were generally residents, only a few years ahead of me, doing the best they could to get their work done and go home. Whatever time they spared for me was to dispense clinical pearls—name the eight causes of a metabolic acidosis or the five causes of a low oxygen level. The attendings lectured us two, maybe three times a week, always about some aspect of physiology and disease. Never about the suffering.

My fellow students were equally distressed. But we were so busy and flabbergasted by what was happening around us that we didn't have time to process our emotions or support one another. We would whiz by each other on the wards with our various teams, a nervous wave the only acknowledgment of our distress. If I ever felt overwhelmed by the sadness or squeamish about the effects of disease on the human body, I had two choices: be the caricature of the medical student, who cries, faints, or vomits— or be silent. I stuck with the latter.

Following medical school, my residency in Boston provided no reprieve from the emotional distress. But now I was in demand for my emerging medical skills as well as the administrative responsibilities required of any resident. My pager buzzed constantly. Nurses fired questions at me whenever I showed my face on the ward. And as the main medical contact for families with the medical team, my sense of inadequacy was no longer about inexperience but about lack of time. I liked this kind of inadequacy a whole lot more. Everyone wanted more of me. Every third day I received ten to twelve new patients on my service. I would spend two days processing them, stabilizing some and discharging others, only to receive twelve more patients on the third day. My scarce free time was largely spent sleeping. It felt as if there was no time to address more than the immediate physiologic needs of my patients.

And this didn't change much during my subspecialty training, or fellowship, in pulmonary and critical care in San Francisco. By this point, I had stopped expecting it would. There was still no time for the open-ended questions I'd been taught to ask in the first two years of medical school. In my pulmonary clinic, where I followed patients over time, I could not seem to connect with them in any depth. These patients were usually scheduled in twenty-minute blocks. Half of them had serious illnesses that put them at severe risk of death and thus of being placed on life support. And for many, that life support would become permanent, accompanying them like a metal straitjacket toward the Great Beyond.

But they didn't seem to realize it. And I had no idea how to tell them. They dutifully showed up for their appointments, many with oxygen tanks in tow, bags of inhalers ready for review. They were coming to me for help, for support, for hope. It felt almost cruel to say that the end was approaching, that I thought it unlikely they would survive another hospitalization, that I was concerned they would die on a breathing machine. I didn't have the time nor did I know the words. I didn't have any alternative options to offer besides more treatment. And I wanted to show them I cared, to have them like me. And so our limited time was spent discussing what I was going to do for them or to them. And my ICU patients, or more often the family members acting as their surrogates, seemed similarly unaware that the end might be approaching. They asked about next steps and other treatment options. They watched monitors or followed lab values. But they expected me to *do something*, which is exactly what I had been trained to do.

And there was always something more to do, something else to try. The protocols that I crammed into my exhausted brain were always about escalating care, designed to guide me through increasing the levels of pharmacologic and technical support. I never even considered that a dying patient might choose comfort as his priority and thus require a protocol to de-escalate the life-prolonging treatments that we steadily heaped on. Moreover, in the frenzy of a medical code, there are so many things to do to keep the heart beating, so many procedures to try, that it was almost inconceivable to waste time investigating whether the person even wanted to be kept alive at all costs.

It was an unspoken rule that we were to resuscitate coding patients until they were almost in rigor mortis, sticking large catheters into every possible orifice, trying everything to keep them alive. The high-adrenaline atmosphere spurred us on. I saw patient after patient meet his end while being prodded with needles and lines by ICU residents eager to learn and to impress.

Often in these cases, everyone in that room knew that the patient would never make it out; we may have known it for days prior. And yet we plowed on, inserting lines and shouting commands until our higher-ups gave us permission to stop. The assumption was always that more was better.

And it wasn't lost on me that, at least in those days, the attendings who were trained in the "doing" subspecialties, like surgery, cardiology, and ICU medicine, seemed to be the heroes. They had the best cars in the parking lot and the best offices in the building. Like my father, they got the most gifts at Christmastime. And we trainees rewarded them too, giving them the highest ratings as teachers and passing on stories about their feats of greatness.

Mastering procedures was the pinnacle of medical training. See one, do one, teach one is the mantra in ICUs, where procedures are divided up among the inexperienced interns by the more senior residents or fellows. The goal is to be assigned a procedure that you haven't done before, learn how to do it step by step from another trainee, and then teach it to someone coming after you. Each resident has to be "signed off" on these procedures by the attending, and like a collector's baseball cards, a great deal of pride is taken in their accumulation. But while there are sign-offs for all kinds of technological procedures, there are none for end-of-life conversations. Or the critical act of breaking bad news through family conferences. And for this reason, many residents consider these communication skills inessential, as did I.

And so with all of this focus on *doing,* we behaved as though death were optional or nonexistent. I avoided talking to families about their loved ones' conditions and instead brought them new treatment options. Both in the clinic and in the ICU. As a parent looking back, it reminds me of the times I bribed a child with

EXTREME MEASURES

candy or television because I was too tired to engage with her. When I entered an ICU room with a dying patient, instead of acknowledging the sadness and the fear, I focused on the catheter kit. As I bustled around the room setting up the procedure, unwrapping the sterile box like a new piece of furniture from IKEA, I saw hope in the patient's face. I had come to do something for her. It couldn't be too bad. And I almost convinced myself it was true.

I looked good on paper—I was working hard, highly skilled, getting paid almost nothing. It was the image I'd always had of myself. The selfless doctor. But I felt spiritually queasy. Something wasn't right, but I lacked the time and support to reflect on what this was. I just felt . . . off.

And so I developed some defense mechanisms. I became inured to the suffering I witnessed every day. I chuckled at the medical students who were still green, knowing it was only a matter of time before they followed my trajectory, repressing their shock and sadness as they shed their naïveté.

Graduating medical students have been reciting the oath of Hippocrates for the past five hundred years. "I will remember," I had recited in 1992, "that there is art to medicine as well as science, and that warmth, sympathy, and understanding may outweigh the surgeon's knife or the chemist's drug." As I said these words, eyes watering, I had no idea how difficult it would be for me to adhere to the oath I was taking.

With the intense focus on curing disease, down to its most esoteric tributaries, using the most sophisticated tools imaginable, I objectified my patients. And this denial is particularly easy in the ICU. My patients were often comatose, tied down, and sedated. I never had the chance to get to know them as the people they had been, their histories, personalities, and quirks. And so while I gained vast technological knowledge during my training, my spirit—the compassion and humanity I had brought with me to medical school in Cleveland—began to atrophy.

I went into medical school a human being, and I came out a doctor.

All That Glitters

When I think back to my training, learning how to use the pulmonary artery catheter, or "the Swan," was possibly the zenith. Introduced in 1970, it was the poster child of exciting new technologies. Until the Swan's debut, only highly trained cardiologists were given access to the fragile recesses of the heart. Using videoscopic X-rays, or fluoroscopy, they tracked the location of the catheter tip at all times so as to avoid perforating or damaging the heart and blood vessels. This required the use of special lead-lined rooms and trained personnel. But the new Swan-Ganz catheter was different. It did not require an operator to steer it because it "sailed" through the heart on the current of blood, buoyed by an inflatable balloon at its tip. Without the need for fluoroscopy or a specialized room with trained personnel, other physicians saw the catheter as a way to get information—such as heart and circulatory system function—that might help their patients, without having to rely on consultants. And so the love affair between the ICU and the Swan began.

The kit, packaged like a TV dinner, had more shiny needles and compartments than most other catheter kits. Unlike the others, which accessed only blood vessels, the Swan entered the sacred territory of the heart, and therefore required much more preparation and gadgetry. Inserting it was almost a religious experience—physicians were dressed to the nines in full sterile regalia: bouffant caps, face shields, masks, long blue gowns, gloves, and shoe coverings. The room was like an ocean, almost everything including our patient covered in blue sterile drapes. We swabbed the patient's neck, the only body part left visible, three times with Betadine. The sterile kit was unwrapped and waiting on the bedside table, needles lined up, syringes filled with lidocaine and saline. And then, when all was ready, two physicians, one often training the other, bent over the patient at the head of the bed. Others would stand at the entrance to the room, clear of the sterile field, to observe the sacred moment when a doctor would enter a patient's heart. As we threaded the catheter in, we turned up the volume on the monitor so that it beeped with every heartbeat in order to alert us to any change in rhythm, which might foretell a dangerous arrhythmia. When the tip of the catheter had finally passed out of the right side of the heart into the pulmonary artery, its resting place, we all breathed a sigh of relief.

Placing a Swan-Ganz catheter became so common that the procedure was honored with its own conjugable verb in medicalese: "I swan, you swan." At the height of its use, the catheter was routinely being inserted in 20 to 40 percent of all ICU patients and annual costs for the procedure exceeded $2 billion.

In 1991, I was first instructed in the use of the Swan by Alfred Connors, the attending during my critical care clerkship in my fourth year of medical school. The honor of working with him in the trenches, with his mix of enthusiasm, intelligence, and compassion, probably counts as one of the reasons I chose to pursue a career in critical care medicine.

He was masterful with the Swan. Under his tutelage, I came to believe in the benefits and elegance of the catheter. But, as it would turn out, it didn't help patients at all. And in an ironic twist, the man who ultimately debunked the Swan was my very own Dr. Connors.

In the summer of 1996, at the peak of the Swan-Ganz's use, I had just begun my pulmonary and critical care fellowship at the University of California, San Francisco. At the time, I was swanning patients left and right. It was in September that the story broke: The Swan wasn't helping and was, in fact, harming patients. The study was published in the reputable *Journal of the American Medical Association*, and there was no ignoring it. When I realized that Dr. Connors was first author on the study, I felt disbelief, maybe a bit of abandonment, and certainly anger—not at Dr. Connors specifically but at the sense that aspersions were being cast on one of the grandest weapons in my arsenal.

Of course, we knew the procedure was dangerous. The catheter often triggered arrhythmias, which were sometimes fatal. But we had convinced ourselves that the risk was worth the benefit, given the helpful information it provided us.

When the news came out, the entire pulmonary and critical care community was up in arms. My colleagues and I felt we were being stripped of one of our great offerings. The study was attacked; the author was attacked. Subsequent studies determined that the numbers we assiduously pulled from the catheter to guide our treatment plan were fool's gold: often inaccurate, incorrectly interpreted, and prompting treatments that themselves worsened patient outcomes. Moreover, we learned that the Swan actually increased the odds of death by 24 percent. Over the ensuing years, more studies followed, demonstrating at best no benefit and at worst increased mortality. A firestorm raged in the medical literature for years afterward. But over time, as the hubbub began to die down, more physicians began to admit that the risk of the procedure was probably not worth the benefit. Today I rarely see the procedure used. Yet the allure is so great that even last month, almost twenty years after its obituaries were written, I found dozens of recently made YouTube videos demonstrating how to insert a Swan-Ganz catheter.

IN AN IRONY THAT I realized only much later, Dr. Connors's study damning the Swan-Ganz catheter was part of a much larger study that was the first to challenge the way end-of-life care was delivered in America. The SUPPORT Trial, published in 1996 and sponsored by the Robert Wood Johnson Foundation, was conducted by a group of physicians concerned about the rise in overly mechanized and painful deaths, many of which occurred in the intensive care unit. And one of the lead investigators in this group was none other than Dr. Alfred Connors, my mentor and inspiration for a career in ICU medicine.

SUPPORT was designed as a two-phase study. Phase I aimed to describe the state of end-of-life care in America. During Phase II, the investigators performed an intervention aimed at improving the findings from Phase I by enhancing communication and information transfer between physician and patients. The results were dismaying on both counts.

Too often, patients were dying in the ICU, in unfamiliar and frightening surroundings, isolated from their families. In the late 1980s and early 1990s, more than 40 percent of deaths occurred in hospitals. More than half the patients who died in hospitals were reported to have moderate to severe pain at least half of the time. Almost 40 percent of patients who died spent at least ten days in an ICU, and 46 percent of those received mechanical ventilation within three days of death. Communication between patients and their doctors about preferences around dying was dismal— for patients who did not want to receive cardiopulmonary resuscitation, only 47 percent of their doctors were aware of this critical piece of information.

There was much hope placed on the SUPPORT Phase II intervention. The hypothesis was that if the study team provided doctors with daily estimates of their patients' prognoses and facilitated communication between the physicians and their patients, medical care would become more closely aligned with the patients' values rather than with the physicians' assumptions. Presumably, this would result in decreased use of nonbeneficial treatments and the accompanying suffering.

Phase II was a complete failure. Despite this intensive intervention, nothing changed. Doctors were no more likely to know their patients' cardiopulmonary resuscitation (CPR) preferences. Patients still died as frequently in ICUs and on breathing machines. And there was no improvement in pain management.

Somehow I didn't hear about this critical study during the entire course of my training, despite the fact that it made its debut at the time that I was training to become an ICU doctor, positioned to manage some of the worst of these deaths. I found out about it only ten years later, in 2006, when I began to pursue training in the burgeoning palliative care movement, for which the study's report was considered essential reading.

It turns out that the SUPPORT study was conducted right under my nose during medical school. Only five sites were chosen, and Dr. Connors's MetroHealth medical center, where I rotated as a student on the ICU service, was one of these. He and his team were gathering data for SUPPORT while I was enthusiastically learning how to prolong life in the ICU. No one, not even the SUPPORT investigators themselves, had any idea how bad the state of death and dying in America was until the data were analyzed and presented in 1996, by which time I was already a critical care fellow.

I recently reached out to Dr. Connors to learn more. I was intrigued and inspired by this man who had been at the center of two groundbreaking trials with powerful implications for both the ICU and my own practice. I imagined that it had taken a lot of courage for him to expose these major problems in the culture to which he had pledged his professional allegiance.

Dr. Connors described the initial shock, even outrage, in the critical care community in reaction to his message about the Swan-Ganz catheter. "When the data were presented at the Society of Critical Care Medicine, you could have heard a pin drop," he told me. He began to feel like a persona non grata. One invitation to participate on a panel about the Swan was abruptly rescinded. Another time, a prominent pulmonologist recommended that he be stripped of his membership in the American Thoracic Society, pulmonary medicine's most prestigious professional organization. Several times he was accosted by angry doctors at national meetings, who felt that he was removing one of their most effective tools. "It is inconceivable for me to manage a critically ill patient with a heart that's not working well without this instrument," the president of the Society of Critical Care Medicine told the *Wall Street Journal*. He compared it to a pilot making a transatlantic flight with only a compass for navigation. The president went on to state that his critical care practice would "continue to confidently use" the Swan-Ganz catheter.

Dr. Connors's response in the same article read: "Knowing that something should work isn't the same as knowing it does work. We shouldn't make these decisions on gut feelings, but on data."

This is so true. But doctors, like other mortals, are driven by many factors besides reason. And our infatuation with the Swan, although proven after twenty-five years to be wrongheaded, is a telling example of how gravely we can mislead ourselves. I view Dr. Connors's willingness to stand tall against such collective conviction as heroic.

I was even more impressed by his role as a lead investigator in the SUPPORT study. Here, instead of focusing on a single, albeit central, intervention, he was questioning the entire system and its culture. What, I asked him, had led him to do that?

His story showed me that while we still have a long way to go, we have already come a great distance in our management of patients at the end of life. In the early 1980s, he told me, Dr. Connors had cared for a patient with advanced emphysema who developed respiratory failure after a surgical procedure. He worked assiduously to keep the patient alive, using every trick in the book—expertly fine-tuning the ventilator (breathing machine), aggressively treating pneumonia, and ordering strong nebulizer treatments in various combinations. However, the patient was very weak and failed all attempts to wean him from the ventilator. He was heavily sedated, which is the case for many patients with temporary breathing tubes passing through their mouths into their lungs. A confused or panicked patient might inadvertently dislodge the tube, which would be disastrous. Following standard procedure, two weeks later Dr. Connors, after obtaining consent from the patient's family, asked the surgeons to "trach" his patient—that is, to insert a tracheostomy tube through his neck, which would replace the temporary breathing tube with a more stable and more permanent connection to the ventilator.

With the trach in place and the patient stabilized following the surgery, the patient's sedation was lowered. Over the next several days, he began to wake up and understand his condition. He watched as courses of antibiotics came and went, one inhaler treatment was substituted for another, and diuretic medicines were given to "dry his lungs out," but the result was the same. He couldn't breathe on his own. And, it turned out, it wasn't how he wanted to live.

He began to beg the medical team to allow him to die. He

scribbled notes, insisting that they disconnect his trach tube from the breathing machine. He mouthed the words to anyone who would listen, squeezing their hands tightly. This was a first for Dr. Connors, who had never before had a patient dependent on life support insist on being released from it. He imagined that the patient didn't understand what would happen. "You will almost certainly die if we remove this machine. Are you sure about this?" The patient remained adamant.

Dr. Connors approached the patient's daughters to discuss this unusual predicament. Over the previous weeks, they had often expressed their appreciation to him for keeping their father alive. So they were surprised to hear him questioning the apparent victory. "I feel bad," he told them. "I don't think we are doing the right thing. I don't think that your father wants us to keep him attached to these machines." At first stunned, they soon regrouped and insisted on continued life prolongation, stating that their father simply wasn't thinking straight. But the patient continued his protest, and Dr. Connors began to realize that he was forcing treatment on this man against his will. Conflict arose. Hospital counsel was put on alert, just in case.

Dr. Connors realized that he needed support. He discussed the case with Stuart Youngner, a psychiatrist at one of the other Cleveland hospitals. Dr. Youngner, who taught my medical school bioethics module, was one of a small number of doctors at the time who had an interest in end-of-life decision making. In our seminars, he presented cases that dealt with the issues that I am most concerned about today: withdrawal of care, family–physician conflict, complex decision making. I am embarrassed to say that I did not pay much attention at the time; I was more interested in the physiology lectures.

Dr. Youngner recommended that Dr. Connors bring the family's priest into the process, as this was a religious family with great trust in their clergy. He suggested that Dr. Connors excuse any nurses from direct care of this patient if they were uncomfortable with the concept of removing life support, which many were. In those days, Dr. Connors told me, very few nurses, and even fewer doctors, were comfortable with the idea of removing a patient from a ventilator knowing he would not be able to breathe on his own. There was concern that this was euthanasia, and it just wasn't done.

After three weeks of ongoing communication in multiple family meetings, the patient's daughters finally agreed to honor their father's request. After talking with the priest, the sisters were able to resolve their fears that they would be complicit in their father's death or acting against God's will. The daughters' trust in Dr. Connors was slowly rebuilt, and the patient's preferences took primacy.

The family gathered around the patient's bed. The team then disconnected his trach from the breathing machine. He lived another sixteen hours, saying his good-byes and holding their hands, then peacefully slipped into his death.

It was this experience that primed Dr. Connors to join the SUPPORT study seven years later. When he first learned about the study's aim, which was to "improve care for seriously ill hospitalized patients," he got chills. He vowed to himself that he would host one of the study sites, as indeed he ultimately did. But although he had concerns about how the health care system was managing dying patients, Dr. Connors could never have conceived of the extent of the problem until the results of SUPPORT were tallied.

FOLLOWING THE DISTURBING RESULTS of SUPPORT, the Robert Wood Johnson Foundation began another phase of study. Promoting Excellence in End-of-Life Care was a national program created in 1997 with the intention of bringing palliative care techniques into the treatment of the dying. Ira Byock, a palliative care physician who served as the director of this program, noticed that many of the 678 letters of intent for the Promoting Excellence grants demonstrated that the field of critical care was ripe for challenge and change. And so, in 1999, Promoting Excellence decided to go right to the belly of the beast, the ICU.

A work group consisting of physician and nurse thought leaders from the critical and palliative care worlds was convened. In the spring of 2002, the program issued a request for proposal (RFP) for an initiative entitled Promoting Palliative Care Excellence in Intensive Care, whose goal was to integrate palliative approaches into mainstream critical care. Of the 242 resulting applications, only four institutions were awarded grants, which they received in March 2003. Among these were the Massachusetts General Hospital, Lehigh Valley Hospital and Health Network, University of Washington Schools of Medicine and Nursing, and the University of Medicine and Dentistry of New Jersey (UMDNJ). I was hired as a critical care physician at UMDNJ in May of 2003, two months after this program was initiated. Thus I was serendipitously given another front-row seat at another attempt by the Robert Wood Johnson Foundation to change the way we care for the dying in this country. This time, though, I would be paying attention. Nurse Pat Murphy, who threatened to call the police on me mere months into my tenure, made sure of it.

ANNE MOSENTHAL AND PAT MURPHY, the UMDNJ's physician–nurse dyad on the Promoting Excellence grant, were a force to be reckoned with. Anne Mosenthal was a trauma–critical care surgeon with an interest in palliative care. And Pat was Pat. Like me, Anne had been practicing in the "life-prolongation at all costs" paradigm of care until she became Pat's mentee in the late 1990s. In 2000, the pair was selected to participate in the Project on Death in America, which helped seed the nascent palliative care movement. The project was the brainchild of Kathleen Foley, a neurologist at Memorial Sloan Kettering Cancer Center in New York City who had been interested for years in the management of cancer pain. It was funded by the Open Society Institute, a nonprofit foundation created by philanthropist George Soros, who would go on to spend $50 million between 1994 and 2003 to support individuals and institutions in overcoming barriers to providing compassionate care to the dying. And in what I have found to be an almost ubiquitous phenomenon among philanthropists in this field, Mr. Soros's commitment was inspired by his own parents' less-than-optimal death experiences.

Anne and Pat's interviewers at the Open Society Institute were very enthusiastic to meet them. Trauma surgeons and nurses were not their usual customers. They expressed amazement when Anne described the protocols of a typical trauma unit. There, patients who were thought likely to remain dependent on machinery for an extended period of time were fitted with a percutaneous endoscopic gastrostomy tube (PEG), a Greenfield (vascular) filter, and a tracheostomy tube (trach), usually within a few days of admission.

A PEG tube is a feeding tube that is surgically inserted through the abdominal wall directly into the stomach. Like the trach, it replaces a temporary tube that had entered the body through the mouth or nose, providing a more stable connection to life-sustaining treatments, in this case artificial nutrition. A Greenfield filter is a barrier that is inserted into the large vein that brings blood up from the legs to prevent blood clots from reaching the heart—a dangerous, often fatal occurrence after surgery, especially in patients for whom medical blood thinning is contraindicated.

In many trauma ICUs at that time, this triad was ordered for every patient deemed likely to require life support for more than three days. This made for safer and more efficient transfers to non-ICU beds when the time came; part of the inherent processes of top-level trauma units. For young trauma patients who would likely recover down the line, the interventions made sense. But for the frail, the chronically diseased, and the dying, such devices tethered the patients to machines, placing them squarely in the path of a mechanized death.

With Anne's description of this triad of treatment, jaws dropped around the table. Pat says it dawned on her at that point that they were a likely shoo-in for Mr. Soros's program, given their status as the first team working with trauma patients to demonstrate interest in this program. And she was right.

Thus two years later they were primed to apply for the Robert Wood Johnson Palliative Care Excellence in Intensive Care grant. Their proposal was to create an interdisciplinary team, called the Family Support Team, consisting of nurses, social workers, and counselors. The goals were to enhance communication, family support, and staff education and to address unmanaged pain or distress. This team was a direct forerunner of UMDNJ's palliative care services, but in 2003, the words *palliative care* were not in the general medical lexicon. The American Board of Medical Specialties wouldn't recognize it as an official subspecialty for three more years.

I met the Family Support Team two months after their grant began. This team went where they felt they were needed, not where we doctors thought they should go. We didn't believe we needed their help. They didn't ask us for permission to talk to our patients, which was unusual and off-putting. They joined our rounds, pulled us aside to ask questions, and engaged with the patients when they felt they needed to. They were tough and unafraid of speaking their minds. Where other nurses I knew might be reticent about their opinions, those on the Family Support Team would come right out and criticize our management of a patient. They would usually find the resident or intern to berate but were equally happy taking me to task.

Pat's team inserted itself into our ICU in a way that I have never seen a palliative care team do since, with confidence and a hint of self-righteousness. And that was what it took for me. Someone brave enough to hold a mirror right up to my face. Looking back, I believe I needed to be hit over the head with a baseball bat by a slugger like Pat to dislodge my inculcated beliefs.

While I initially resented Pat, I came to welcome her, even seek her out, when struggling with a case. She taught me how to use the word *dying* with my patients or their families. She showed me that patients wouldn't roll over and become hysterical but would often be appreciative, even relieved, to hear what they somehow knew was true. She taught me how to sit with raw grief and emotion by counting slowly to ten. She also taught me to forgive myself if my patient died.

I don't remember who told me to read up on the SUPPORT study, but likely it was Pat. "What? You haven't read the SUPPORT study? Where've you been? Go read it right now," is what she would have said. By then I was ready to follow Pat and the Family Support Team right to the center of the palliative care movement.

THE WORD *PALLIATIVE* COMES FROM the Latin word *palliare*, "to cloak." This protective gesture poetically communicates the intent behind the relatively new specialty of palliative care. The discipline gained traction in the 1980s in the United States, but usually in the context of patients receiving hospice care during the AIDS crisis. And although it achieved more recognition after the publication of the SUPPORT study in 1996, most clinicians, including myself, would not hear of it until much later.

Palliative care is an interdisciplinary approach to managing suffering in the context of medical illness, whether physical, emotional, familial, or spiritual. Social workers, chaplains, nurses, and physicians work collaboratively to attend to the needs of the whole patient rather than just her failing organs. Communication is a central tenet of the specialty. Palliative care isn't only for the dying: any patient with serious symptoms or communication needs can benefit. But for patients approaching the end of life, its offerings are often critical.

When I first heard of it, this holistic approach to patient care was already familiar to a small number of specialties, such as geriatrics, family medicine, and primary care. But it was anathema in the ICU. Yet under Pat's tutelage, I began to see how critical these skills were to ICU practice. Our technologies carry far more potential burdens than the tools of geriatricians. And so I realized that it was essential that our technical offerings be tempered by consideration of the whole patient, not just her organ function.

A generic explanation of the risks of a procedure—required in exchange for a signature on a consent form—was a poor substitute for clarifying the true benefits, and the burdens, of a treatment. And we rarely acknowledged the bigger picture: that the patient might be dying.

And to my surprise, following these deeper conversations, many patients opted out of the treatments I'd assumed they would want. I learned to step back from my "do everything" instinct and pause. I worked to tease out the most important requirements and then to honor them, which sometimes meant avoiding treatments that once were so reflexive. I came to see that in our zeal to save life, we often worsened death.

Once my eyes had been opened to the suffering we could inflict, I saw it everywhere. For many, the ICU functions as an antechamber of death. It is often the final stage in what I have come to call the "end-of-life conveyor belt," where dying patients are hoisted onto what I imagine as a moving platform, receiving protocolized treatments to prop up their failing organs. For such patients, this conveyor belt moves inexorably toward a predictable destination in a pattern that has grown grimly familiar to me. By the time the patient dies, he is encased in life support, arms tied down to prevent accidental dislodgement of tubes, unable to eat, talk, or escape—other than through death.

Let me qualify. I'm a big advocate of life support in the appropriate context. It is why I went into critical care. I recently cared for a thirty-year-old man whose heart had stopped while he was playing pick-up basketball. He came to us almost dead and would certainly have died without our aggressive use of life support. Three days after his admission, he went home to resume his life. And it is not only for the young. Our technology recently benefited an eighty-five-year-old woman with a urinary tract infection who arrived at our ICU critically ill and in profound shock. She was restored by our use of antibiotics, fluids, and blood pressure support medications to her baseline, albeit frail, health. And went back home to her family. The metaphor of an end-of-life conveyor belt applies only to those patients for whom our technologies will obviously not help—those who are dying.

Along with showing me the need for responsible use of these powerful technologies, palliative care also opened my eyes to the pain I had learned to inure myself against. And then taught me what to do about it.

Of course we treated pain in the ICU. But we thought of it as an on–off switch. If there was pain, we started an opioid drip. But it often wasn't well calibrated or carefully assessed. Sometimes the patient was so overmedicated, it might take days for him to wake up. Other times, my patients were undertreated for pain, or worse, on sedative medications that don't treat pain at all but keep patients quiet, so I might not even realize they were suffering.

And because our top priority was maintaining blood pressure and organ function, pain management, with its medications that might lower blood pressure, came in second. Even now, with all of my palliative care training, I still wince when I write an order to start pain or sedation medications on a patient who has very low blood pressure. I do it, but it goes against everything I was originally taught.

With Pat's coaching, I realized that I treated pain only in those who were writhing or grimacing or who had obvious indications, like a recent surgery or trauma. But subtler cases passed me by. And other non-pain symptoms, such as agitation, delirium, constipation, or anxiety, usually fell completely by the wayside.

I had also been taught to hold off on treating certain types of pain until the consulting physician, usually a surgeon or neurologist, had examined the patient. The thinking was that if pain was diminished by medication, the surgeon might lose valuable diagnostic information on her clinical exam. And for those patients whose neurological status was unclear, we believed that pain management should occur only after a neurologist or neurosurgeon had performed an assessment, lest the patient be too sleepy to participate in the exam. And thus I often delayed or withheld pain medications from patients who needed them. In addition, treating pain almost felt as though we were accepting that it might be here to stay. That felt like failure.

It took the palliative care movement to teach me that treating pain early on was one of the most important things I could do for my patients—almost as important as maintaining blood pressure or treating infection. I hadn't understood how prevalent pain was in the ICU, how much suffering patients were experiencing. When I began to imagine myself or a loved one in that bed, I realized that I would want my doctor to prioritize pain management. Moreover, multiple studies have shown that providing patients with analgesia does not compromise diagnosis. I began to understand that simultaneous management of disease and pain was not only doable but also critical, although it took some learning to find my balance. Maybe, I thought, we should have protocols for a Code Pain like we do for Code Blue.

I WAS BECOMING A CONVERT to palliative care. I had seen the error in my ways and was learning that there was a way to make amends. I was devouring research reports and ruminating over the alarming statistics. Over 50 percent of Americans die in pain. Seventy percent die in institutions. And 30 percent of families lose most of their life savings while caring for a dying loved one.

If I weren't already convinced, I then read a study demonstrating that choosing hospice over continued disease-oriented treatment prolonged the lives of patients with several types of life-limiting diseases by an average of a month. Another study a few years later found that patients with serious cancers receiving palliative care consultations in addition to standard care lived longer by an average of two months.

These are the types of statistics, I thought, that make for a revolution.

Vital Decisions

In 2004, Pat introduced me to Helen Blank, a bioethicist teaching at UMDNJ. Helen believed that hospitalized patients with life-limiting illness needed support to tailor treatment options to their own preferences and values. The Chief Medical Officer (CMO) at a local health insurance company shared Helen's philosophy and they made an unusual arrangement. The company would pay Helen and two other colleagues to perform bedside consultations on patients with serious or end-of-life illness.

This was a very brave and unusual decision on the part of the insurance company at that time. The seeds of Sarah Palin's "death panel" hysteria had been sown, and no health care insurer wanted to be seen talking to its patients about the D-word. But the CMO believed in the concept of patient-centered decision making. It was logical. It was ethical. And, he knew from the emerging palliative care literature, it was what patients wanted.

The goal of the consultation would be to enhance the patient's understanding of her diagnosis and prognosis as well as to identify personal values and goals. Armed with more information, personal clarity, and self-confidence, the patient would presumably be more likely to receive medical care that was right for him.

Completing such bedside consults turned out to be extremely difficult. More often than not, the patient would be comatose or at least sleeping when Helen arrived to talk with him. Or the family would have just stepped out of the room.

In an act of courage and ingenuity, the CMO agreed to let Helen and her colleagues conduct their consultations over the phone. And so the floodgates opened. What had been two, maybe three cases a week became five a day. Helen started to panic. How would she and two other part-time counselors handle a potential avalanche of cases? They needed more partners. I was fascinated by the concept, and before I knew it, I had signed on to do these end-of-life telephone consultations. Then, before he knew it, my husband, Mark, an MBA with a background in health care, became our de facto CEO. Vital Decisions was born.

Helen and I spent countless hours developing the first iteration of Vital Decisions' electronic counseling forms. We worked constantly, with the frenzy of a startup and the passion of promoting change. We often worked at my dining room table, where I'd do double duty as a mother of three young children, our work sessions punctuated by the mundane activities of life—lighting Hanukkah candles, drinking coffee (hot or cold depending on the weather), relying on junk food and television to keep my children occupied.

We didn't feel any need to reinvent the wheel and searched high and low to find existing scripts for initiating conversations about advance care planning. But we came up empty. No scripts, no data collection forms, no strategies for beginning to walk through these important topics with frightened and vulnerable strangers. We ended up creating an interview structure that grew organically from our own experience. And over the ensuing years, we were asked repeatedly to lend our material to those coming after us.

Early on, we realized that we needed to go straight to the patient herself, without asking the permission of her doctor, much as Pat's team had done in the ICU. Our medical system is based around a covenantal relationship between a patient and her doctor, which many believe should not be breached. And so Helen and I experienced resistance, or at least disinterest, from physicians when we would request permission to contact their patients. They usually did not call us back, and if they did, they were often suspicious and uncomfortable. It was simply unworkable to give the physicians gatekeeper privileges regarding end-of-life conversations with their patients. So we didn't. I was concerned that there would be a backlash, but there never was. The patients didn't seem concerned that we had not spoken to their physicians first. We were careful never to provide medical advice or criticize a doctor's decisions.

It was a tricky business, cold-calling seriously ill patients to discuss end-of-life issues. We were strangers, referred by the patients' health insurance plan—already a set-up for mistrust. We worried that patients would think we were just trying to save their insurance companies money. On top of that, the patients' doctors were not even involved. In addition, our service was "opt in"—participation was completely voluntary. We didn't expect many people to want to take our call.

We were astonished by the response. In our introductory script, we explained that just as cardiologists focused on the heart, our expertise lay in the medical decision-making process. And, apparently, they wanted what we were offering. Once we reached them by telephone, most patients were not only willing but eager to speak to us. They seemed to be aching for information and support. Very few patients had any idea what their doctors were thinking and most had no idea how to ask. Many didn't realize that their illness was life limiting and were baffled by their deteriorating functional status in the face of continued treatment. Often they felt alone, bewildered, and terrified. We offered patients the support they needed to articulate their wishes and ensure that those preferences were communicated to family members and providers so that ultimately they would be honored.

We received our referrals from the health plans' case managers. Helen and I arranged "road shows" where we would drive to various offices to introduce ourselves to the case managers. We presented them with lists of diseases and social situations that could be red flags, such as metastatic cancer, serious family discord in the face of life-limiting illness, and long hospital stays. We described how we could help in these cases. It often felt as if we were traveling saleswomen, exhibiting our wares in the hopes that case managers would see their value and actually use them. When referral rates started to sag, we hit the road again.

In those days of the early 2000s, almost no one had heard of palliative care. Helen and I joked that we had to spell out the word *palliative* multiple times per day. And if we mentioned the word *hospice,* we were often met by silence or discomfort on the other end of the phone. *Hospice*—a philosophy of care that uses palliative care principles with patients approaching the end of life—had a serious marketing problem. To laypeople, it meant the end of the line, no more hope. To physicians, it signaled personal failure— an admission that they couldn't keep the patient alive. But once we explained to our patients that research demonstrated palliative care and hospice almost always improved quality of life, usually without shortening it, most were glad to know it existed, even if they were not ready to engage with it at that particular time.

With practice, Helen and I became increasingly skilled at coaching patients. We learned to ask more than tell, to sit with the sadness and despair of patients and their families, and to acknowledge uncertainty. The data we collected and the surveys we administered over the next few years proved that patients and their family members appreciated our service and ultimately made different medical decisions as a result of it—like choosing hospice more frequently than similar patients who had not gone through our program.

I moved on to other endeavors in 2012, but the service is still going strong. By 2016, Vital Decisions had counseled tens of thousands of patients and family members, with plans to help another 15,000 during that year.

Helping create that company taught me more about patient-centered care than medical school, residency, and fellowship put together.

As medical director of Vital Decisions in 2008, I felt it was important to get my stripes in palliative care. This was the first year that the American Board of Internal Medicine would recognize palliative care as a legitimate specialty. It is common for new boards to allow experienced practitioners without formal fellowship training to be "grandfathered" into the community after passing the board exam. And so with Pat as my sponsor, I went on to become certified in the new field of hospice and palliative care medicine.

In 2009, after seven years in New Jersey, my family returned to the San Francisco Bay area. Serendipitously, one of the palliative care physicians at the University of California, San Francisco (UCSF) had suddenly gone out on medical leave. The team needed coverage—and fast. And so I would spend my first year as a card-carrying palliative care physician at the same place where I had trained, a decade and a half earlier, in pulmonary and critical care medicine. As I prepared for my first week of work as a palliative care attending, I imagined how now, instead of single-mindedly working to prolong life, I would use the skills I'd cultivated over the previous years to help patients choose the treatment plan that most closely aligned with their preferences and values. Much as I had run through my Code Blue protocols as a young intern, I now ran through my protocols for treating the symptoms that often accompany dying and disease—pain, cough, itching, nausea—those I had once considered of secondary importance. Now, instead of rushing through the halls with the code team, I would provide patients with a completely different kind of support.

It would ultimately prove to be a redemptive experience, to walk these same halls with an entirely new set of skills, to broaden my offerings to patients. But I got off to a humbling start. My third consult as a palliative care attending at UCSF would serve to teach me that even with both critical and palliative care toolboxes at my disposal, caring for patients at the end of life wasn't necessarily going to be easy.

Straddling Two Worlds

When I set eyes on the patient in room 1407, my first thought was, *This lady needs to be intubated, stat!*

The only trouble, I thought to myself, *was that I had been consulted to help ease this patient's passing, not to prolong her life.*

An hour earlier, the team had told me that Mrs. Z, an eighty-two-year-old widow, was dying from pneumonia and did not want to be put on life support. *What a change of pace,* I thought as I hung up the phone. Too often, as an intensivist, I was tasked with keeping dying ICU patients alive. Here I was being asked to honor an elderly woman's request to die in peace.

By now I had learned how to palliate respiratory distress, even without the use of a breathing machine. Some morphine to ease the shortness of breath, a quiet environment, perhaps a touch of antianxiety medicine and a gentle fan. I had other options available, depending on the particular condition causing the shortness of breath.

But it wasn't going to be that simple.

Mrs. Z, a beautiful woman who bore a striking resemblance to Anne Bancroft, somehow remained elegant even in her distress. Her hair had clearly been "done" right before her admission, with only the lock that now strayed in front of her bluish lips out of order.

As I leafed through her chart, I was astonished to find a surprisingly benign medical history: she'd suffered no real medical problems until a few days back, when she'd been brought to the emergency room for a bowel obstruction. At that time, nothing was passing through and she'd been vomiting violently for several hours. Over the next three days, while the bowel obstruction was clearing up, pneumonia had blossomed from the fluid she had aspirated into her lungs.

Now I noted Mrs. Z's blue lips and rapid breathing. She was delirious from lack of oxygen, mumbling incoherently. This was not good.

A Filipino woman sat at the bedside, crying softly. I introduced myself and asked, "How do you know Mrs. Z?"

In faltering English, she explained that she had been Mrs. Z's housekeeper for the past eight years. When Mr. Z had died three years ago, she had moved into the home at Mrs. Z's request.

"She was all alone. Lonely. When he died, she had no children, no friends. She was always so sad and didn't want to talk much. I tried to cheer her up, but . . ." She shrugged sadly, then lifted up Mrs. Z's forearm and pointed to a line of numbers tattooed on the inner side.

My heart dropped. This woman was a Holocaust survivor. She looked like my grandmother. I felt a primal instinct to save her—from what, I wasn't sure.

And I didn't yet know the half of it.

Scanning Mrs. Z's chart, I learned that she had been imprisoned at Auschwitz, where she had fallen victim to Dr. Mengele's insane "experiments" conducted on twins. He had removed her uterus, leaving her with embarrassing abdominal disfigurement and intermittent small-bowel obstructions for which she had been hospitalized many times. Her twin sister had perished at the butcher's hands, and she had been the only member of her extended family to survive the Holocaust. She had married another survivor after the war, and they had eventually made it to safety in America. Her husband's death had left her childless and alone.

A firestorm was raging in my head. Pneumonia is treatable. With immediate intubation to support her breathing, maybe we could turn things around.

But wait. I had been called to the bedside to provide palliative care, not intensive care.

Palliative care is generally expected to lower medical aggressiveness, not raise it. Here and now, I might singlehandedly reverse that trend. Not a good move, I thought, on my first day at the job.

I called the patient's primary medical team and we huddled together outside her room.

"She got worse this morning," the young attending explained, "so I told her that she could either have a tube placed down her throat and go to the ICU, or go to the palliative care suite and be comfortable. She wanted to be comfortable."

"But do you really think she understood?" I asked, trying my best not to sound judgmental. Another role of the palliative care team is to support the doctors caring for the patients in the trenches. I felt I might be on the verge of messing that up now as well. "She has high CO_2 levels; she's confused. Also, she's a Holocaust survivor. She's probably terrified of anyone doing anything to her. Maybe we should just sedate her and intubate."

Clearly, the team found my words distressing. At the beginning of her hospitalization, when the patient had still been alert, the team's focus had been on treating her pneumonia. As she had continued to get sicker, they had tried harder, adjusting antibiotics, increasing the frequency of breathing treatments. But they hadn't actually talked with her about what to do if things didn't go as they all hoped. And when the team was finally compelled to engage with her on this difficult question, she was no longer fully present. And so her rejection of the breathing tube, even though she was disoriented at the time, was all they had to go on. They determined that she preferred the path of comfort management over life prolongation. The morphine they'd administered had eased Mrs. Z's shortness of breath. She was quieter, more peaceful than before, and they were feeling relieved. They had called me, as a palliative care specialist, to support their decision and enhance her comfort. But I was just making it harder.

"I'm just not comfortable intubating her," said the attending. "I feel like she was awake enough to understand me when she made her decision."

There was some murmuring.

"I'm not completely sure she really got it," a respiratory therapist at the back of the gathering crowd piped up. "She was pretty out of it."

"Look," said the young attending, "I spent a lot of time with her, I did the best I could to persuade her, and she really didn't want the tube. I would feel like I was going against her wishes if she got intubated."

"Would you consider trying a BiPAP mask overnight?" I asked. These masks are strapped tightly to a patient's nose and mouth, providing pressurized air to support inhalation. This may work well enough to allow a patient to avoid a breathing tube. But this treatment is recommended only for patients who are alert and not very sick, as this type of mask can be uncomfortable and scary, or just plain dangerous for an inadequately monitored patient—it might slip off, or the patient might vomit into it and aspirate. I knew the risks, but within the constraints of what had already been decided, it seemed like a compromise worth making. We might be able to save this woman's life.

And so I rushed off to the ICU to request a bed for the patient.

While we often put patients on BiPAP on the hospital floor, given this patient's status at this point, the ICU's higher nurse-to-patient ratio would add an extra level of support. Entering my old stomping grounds, I came upon one of the physicians who had taught me during my fellowship. He was the attending in the ICU that day. It had been ten years since I'd last seen him, and I explained that I was working there in a completely different capacity. He nodded politely, but when I asked him for a bed for Mrs. Z, he looked perplexed. "But she's DNR [do not resuscitate], isn't she? She doesn't need to be in the ICU." I reminded him of the principle that he himself had taught me, that patients on BiPAP required close nursing care, especially if their mental status was waxing and waning.

"Well," he said, "the emergency room is full. I really can't give up a bed for a patient who doesn't want to be resuscitated." The respiratory therapist from the floor had accompanied me, and as we walked out of the ICU, he said that he would be willing to watch the patient on BiPAP on the floor. "I'll be there most of the night." It wasn't ideal and we both knew it, but there didn't seem to be a choice.

Later that evening, I slunk out of the hospital. Had I made everything worse? Mrs. Z was still short of breath and confused. The team was upset with me. And I was doing something that I'd been trained not to do—use noninvasive ventilation on a patient who wasn't fully alert. And on the regular medical floor. Nothing was right about any of it, and yet it was the best I could come up with.

The next morning, my worst fears were realized. Delirious and terrified, Mrs. Z writhed in the bed, her mask off center and totally ineffective.

"I tried all night to keep her mask on," the nurse told me, "but she keeps pulling it off. She's afraid that she'll suffocate."

I knew that I couldn't save Mrs. Z without full ICU care, and I didn't know if she would even want us to try. In fact, I really didn't know anything about her. Was I projecting my own values onto a patient who might truly prefer to die in comfort? Was I being swayed by her tragic history, living proof of an evil that had scarred my family and community? Saving her might have felt, on some pre-conscious level, like an attempt to right an immeasurable wrong. Were my ICU instincts overpowering me and affecting my ability to remain patient-centered? Whatever my reasons, it was clear in retrospect that my approach had not worked, and had, in fact, made things worse.

I made a decision: I would be a palliative care doctor. I would not increase Mrs. Z's suffering again. I had the expertise to keep her comfortable, and now I would use it without hesitation. I called the palliative care suite. "We have a patient coming up. Please prepare a morphine drip."

Mrs. Z died four hours later, looking comfortable, her hairdo smoothed around her beautiful face.

I will never know if I did the right thing in the case of Mrs. Z, but what I have learned is this: There is seldom one right approach. The team had determined to the best of their abilities that the patient did not wish to be intubated. But in medicine, we tend to be very binary about how to care for patients. It's either a full-court press or comfort care. But mightn't she still have done better in an ICU bed, despite her do-not-resuscitate order, with a dedicated critical care nurse and respiratory therapist to manage her BiPAP? We'll never know.

When I first heard of her, I was relieved that she had not been hoisted onto the end-of-life conveyor belt. But as I came to view it, she had been put onto a different type of conveyor belt, one that closed the doors of intensive care against her. Conveyor belts, regardless of their destination, are not meant for human beings.

My initial years of practice were focused on keeping hearts beating at all costs. Later, I became a disciple of a different approach to care, where a "good death" was the ultimate goal. Yet neither of these, alone, is the answer. The cases that bring me the most pride and satisfaction are those in which I am able to connect with the patient, understand what she wants me to do, and carry it out. Sometimes that results in a full-court approach, other times in a calm death surrounded by family in a palliative care suite. But often it is some combination of the two approaches.

Regardless of the path, it should be guided by the paradigm of patient-centered care. This type of care is driven by what best serves the patient, regardless of the doctor's own training, bias, or personal history. It should not be based on the location of the patient at the time. We should not assume that because someone happens to be in bed 5 of the ICU she would choose to undergo cardiac resuscitation if her heart stopped, or have a catheter placed in her neck when her metastatic cancer entered its final stages. We should not assume that someone's diagnosis of cancer confers a desire to be the recipient of toxic chemotherapies.

Similarly, if a patient's goals of care are primarily about maximizing quality of life, health care teams should not assume that all attempts at curing the underlying disease must be avoided. Mrs. Z was a terribly difficult case—it is hard to know what she would have chosen had she been fully alert and able to make decisions. And despite my discomfort with how it unfolded, I am confident that we all strived to act in her best interests. But clearly it would have been better to understand her preferences around death and dying when she was still able to fully engage with us.

Patient-centered care is how we would all be practicing were we to abide by the Hippocratic oath pledged at our graduations. It should be a grounding principle at the core of every subspecialty in medicine, and within the hearts and minds of all physicians everywhere. It should not be subsumed by the specialty of palliative care but rather housed within the entire culture of medicine, in every medical school, residency program, and fellowship. It has taken practicing at the intersection of two very different philosophies of care—one that tends to prioritize quantity of life, the other, quality—to understand that good medicine is more nuanced than a single approach. It has to be about the patient. Each patient. That learning has made for one hell of a decade.

chapter three

Abandoned in a Sea of Options

MARIAM'S HEADSCARVES WERE GORGEOUS. The fabrics were colorful and threaded through with gold. A resident in our medicine program, she'd come to this country several years earlier after completing medical school in her native Pakistan. Over the previous two years, I had grown close to her and always enjoyed having her on my service. She was smart, diligent, and dependable. Her patient that day was dying, had been for the previous several weeks. What had started out as zealous, pedal-to-the-metal medical care had become a vehicle to prolong the patient's death. And now, more organs were beginning to shut down—today, the patient's kidneys. And yet her family had remained indelibly optimistic despite all of our bad news, broken hesitantly at first and then with increasing bluntness. They believed in miracles, they said, and expected us to keep working full speed ahead until God pulled one out of his hat.

The typical next step for kidney failure is to start hemodialysis, a process in which the patient's blood is cleaned by a machine, in place of the damaged kidneys, several times a week. In order to accomplish this, the patient's blood supply must be accessed by catheters large enough to pass the entire body's blood volume over the course of a few hours. Placement of these catheters is risky, especially for critically ill patients, and painful.

But I pointed out to the team that in this patient's case, dialysis would not impact the underlying disease that was rapidly shutting down her organs. As we discussed it, we agreed that the procedure would not help the patient in any significant way, even though it might temporarily improve her lab values—something that every doctor has been trained to achieve. But in the final analysis, dialysis would only add risk and suffering. Yet given what we knew about the family, we were concerned they would insist on dialysis anyway.

We began to strategize an approach. I suggested that we not bring it up and simply explain that her kidneys had now begun to shut down. If they asked about dialysis, we would stress that it would not be of medical benefit and point out the less risky but less effective treatments we were already using to address the kidney failure. Then I turned to Mariam, the resident primarily in charge of the patient, and asked her how she would approach the family.

She bowed her head with a smile and then looked up. "You really want to hear what I think?"

I nodded. Of course I did.

"No offense, but you Americans make me laugh. We've spent a half hour trying to figure out a way to avoid doing something that it makes no sense to do. In Pakistan, if we don't think that something will help a patient, we wouldn't even consider offering it. And they would never ask for it either. They would trust our judgment."

It was so obvious, and a little embarrassing. But I also felt a spike of pride. I love being from a culture that believes in autonomy, even if we sometimes approach it the wrong way. Since my conversation with Mariam, I've surveyed many residents and colleagues from other countries, and what I've learned is that our approach is far from universal; indeed, it's distinctly American. Our zeal for unimpeded medical access trumps even that of other industrialized countries. In a recent study of seven wealthy, industrialized nations, it was found that in 2010, over 40 percent of Americans dying from cancer were admitted to the ICU in the last six months of life. That figure was more than double any of the other six countries studied. And on average, American patients dying of cancer had twice as many ICU days as similar patients from the other countries studied.

"Not to Abandon"

The way we practice medicine now is an historical aberration. Until the mid-twentieth century, doctors took control of all medical decisions for their patients, a form of medical paternalism. There was an implicit acceptance that they were best equipped by their training and superior knowledge to chart the most appropriate course of action for their patients. Questions weren't usually asked and instructions were carefully heeded by patients.

And physicians upheld their responsibility in this covenantal relationship by refusing to abandon their patients. The 1903 version of the American Medical Association's Code of Medical Ethics states:

The medical attendant ought not to abandon a patient because deemed incurable; for, continued attention may be highly useful to the sufferer, and comforting to the relatives, even in the last period of the fatal malady, by alleviating pain and by soothing mental anguish. (Section 7)

Doctors sat at bedsides with sick patients late into the night. They visited them in their homes, ate meals that their families prepared, and provided a calm and steady presence. They knew their patients well and usually cared for them over large spans of their lives. They tended to be generalists, able to deliver babies, treat illnesses, and minister to the dying. They were not focused, as physicians tend to be today, on only one organ system and its physiology; rather, they cared for the whole patient and his family.

Norman Rockwell captures the American version of this doctor in many of his iconic renderings. Rockwell published 323 original covers for the *Saturday Evening Post*, which today credits his magazine covers with mirroring "cherished American ideals and values." Almost all of the doctors are graying men in their sixties, and they appear sage, patient, and attentive. They sit with children and worried families, hearing their concerns, comforting them by doing all of the doctorly things done in those days: taking a pulse, looking at a thermometer, caring for a little girl's rag doll.

While some view his work as kitschy or bourgeois, his portraits struck a chord for many Americans. Although I'm somewhat embarrassed to admit it, I too am comforted by that nostalgic version of medical culture. When I think of whom I want at my bedside when I'm sick, it is someone with those qualities— someone who knows me well and will sit with me as long as I need, with a watchful, concerned eye.

But that image of the American doctor underwent a drastic

makeover beginning in the 1960s. As hair got longer and skirts got shorter, the demographic of the American doctor changed dramatically. While only 9 percent of students entering medical school in 1965 were women, by 1975, that number was over 20 percent; today, it approaches 50 percent.

Physicians and their patients, once demographically matched, were becoming more foreign to each other. No longer were black patients restricted from receiving care in most white hospitals. Jewish doctors were being granted increased access to mainstream hospitals. Doctors might now look different from their patients, speak different languages, and have different cultural norms in terms of illness, treatment, and communication.

Not only were the players themselves changing, but the power dynamic was too. The women's movement, the quest for civil rights, and the antiwar movement all valued equality and the decentralization of power. And this spirit penetrated the paternalistic world of medicine, fueled by revelations of abuse of power. Nazi doctors, who conducted brutally sadistic acts on mostly Jewish prisoners in the name of research, became a symbol of the potential evils of unfettered and unregulated medicine. And in 1972, the world learned about the egregious experiments at Tuskegee University, a research study conducted by the U.S. Public Health Service spanning forty years. White medical doctors had experimented on syphilis-infected black patients without their knowledge or consent, dispassionately observing them as they deteriorated, and eventually died, from their infections—again, all in the name of medical research. The study would likely have gone on longer had it not been shut down after a leak to the press.

These profound violations of the authority granted physicians for millennia were met with shock and horror and a collective commitment to never again tolerate these violations of personal autonomy. Even the more benign paternalism practiced by old-time doctors no longer sat right. How could such physicians be so sure that an eighty-six-year-old patient with breast cancer wouldn't want to hear the C-word? And thus the traditional power relationship between patient and physician, in which doctors held all of the cards and patients trusted them implicitly, began to crumble.

I HAD PAID LITTLE ATTENTION to bioethics until I started Vital Decisions with Helen Blank. As we sat at my dining room table into the wee hours, sipping cold coffee and finessing our scripts, she gave me a crash course in the bioethics I had been indifferent to in medical school. I learned of the four principles that formed the foundation. *Beneficence* requires that the physician act with the intent of helping the patient, while *nonmaleficence* mandates that the physician avoid harming the patient. *Justice* is applied when the physician or society regulates the distribution of resources in a way that is most beneficial to the entire population. And *patient autonomy* implies that the patient is empowered to make decisions free from coercion.

I learned that there is no hierarchy to these principles; instead the practitioner must balance them in regard to each specific case. For example, it may be impossible to pursue both nonmaleficence and beneficence at the same time in a patient who requires a dangerous surgery to save his life. Classic bioethics requires a balancing of principles to best serve the needs of the patient.

In the roiling latter half of the twentieth century, however, the principle of patient autonomy took primacy over the other three. I would assert that this is because it is the only principle that gives power back to the individual patient; the others depend on the actions of physicians.

In theory, this sounds like a very good move. But in practice, it backfired. The belief that more is better runs deep in this culture, and the prioritization of autonomy translated into handing patients access to all the marketplace had to offer.

Starting in the 1930s, new technologies were being developed at a meteoric rate. They were changing the world in incredible ways, and we bought into them, hook, line, and sinker. It was generally believed that if a treatment existed, it must be helpful. And American consumerism played a role, too. If someone is selling, we're interested. We're adept at hunting down sources of information and opportunity. Indeed, when we are patients, we reach for the best care we can—and these days we are enabled by the Internet: we Google, we Wiki, we read articles from the Mayo Clinic and the Cancer Treatment Centers of America. Some of us have the resources to fly across the country and spend months in specialty housing at a fancy clinic. In my experience, that alluring possibility—of being the one in ten thousand who recovers—also seduces us further into that trap. We all want to be cared for by "the A team," or "the best kidney man," as my grandmother would have said. We want everything we can get.

A typical patient cannot be expected to understand that, in the case of health care, doing more might lead to a worse outcome and more suffering. Most patients, especially dying patients, need the counsel of a trained health care professional who understands the limits of gleaming new technologies. Yet physicians are reticent to speak up for many reasons. First, they themselves were not immune to the "more is better" philosophy. In addition, offering more feels like being a better advocate—it is evident that they are really *trying*.

And doing more is something patients and families, and even medical teams, can understand and rally behind. It represents hope, competence, and confidence all rolled into one. Moreover, a physician's recommendation to reduce the intensity of care may be met with suspicion on the part of the patient or family as if he is just trying to save money. I can attest to the fact that it frequently is. And, of course, there is always the fear of a lawsuit; although I have never been sued, I feel subjectively more vulnerable to a legal challenge when I do less than when I do more. For all these reasons, the physician has taken a back seat when it comes to the decision-making process, lest she appear to be impinging on her patient's autonomy.

And so we have the perfect storm—each of these factors combining to result in a no-holds-barred, full-steam-ahead approach to medical treatment. There are often no discussions about whether to use these treatments, simply informational scripts about potential risks, and these quickly glossed over, as patients almost never reject treatments offered. Unfettered access has become the new medical ethic. And so the focus of the new doctor–patient relationship has become transactional. We are medical vending machines, our treatments arranged behind a piece of glass. Just press D3 and we'll get going. Unto eternity.

AS I SEE IT, there is no clear villain here. Where Rockwell's doctors had seen their patients as people in a wider social context, we modern doctors were trained in silos that focused on the organ, not the organism, the human. It is much easier to continue to treat a particular organ, even if your patient is dying, if you are wearing blinders.

The American Board of Internal Medicine created twenty-one separate medical specialties between 1936 and 2010, each with its own set of complex tools. These paths were not only more financially lucrative than general practice but also provided one with a sense of competence and mastery. Over those years, doctors began to pursue subspecialty training with zeal. In my residency at the Brigham and Women's Hospital, the 1995 graduating class of sixty produced only three primary care physicians, one of whom eventually went on to pursue a specialty in gastroenterology. Like a blind man touching the side of an elephant, doctors began to lose sight of the person at the other end of their stethoscope.

The patient was similarly blinded by the implication that action implied hope. "Do you want us to do everything to save your sister?" Temporarily saving her lungs might not translate into saving her quality of life, but even a well-meaning physician might fail to clarify this. All the fuss and bother focused on maintaining an organ could easily be misinterpreted by a desperate patient or family member as restorative to overall health. The sheer flurry of activity in the room takes on a life of its own, and expecting a patient to say, "Wait a minute, can we talk about this first?" is a tall order.

And it is rarely clear whom to ask. At the end of life, a typical patient tends to have multiple interactions with multiple subspecialists, one for each organ that is failing. A friend with cancer told me that she referred to her oncologist not as her doctor but as her cancer's doctor. Each physician makes specialized recommendations for more treatments. Seldom does one of these procedures rule out another—there's always room for another catheter or drug. And patients simply cannot keep track of who is caring for them. My patients often complain of a virtual revolving door of faces, with doctors coming in and out of their rooms, and no idea who they are or what team they represent. And the numbers of these doctors tend to diminish as they run out of new technologies and treatments to offer.

Consultation etiquette can also serve to keep patients in the dark. In my palliative care role, I am sometimes stymied from presenting the big picture; medical culture dictates that the disease-focused specialists must first weigh in on their treatment recommendations. For example, oncology consultations are usually triggered automatically for hospitalized patients with cancer diagnoses, even if the patient is so critically ill that chemotherapy is unlikely to help.

But hospice services, which provide palliative care interventions to patients either in their homes or in nursing facilities and which have been shown to be of great benefit to patients with cancer, are not available to those receiving disease-focused treatments such as chemotherapy. Yet instead of presenting these two options at the same time and letting the patient choose between them, there is a clear hierarchy to the usual medical protocol. The decision about chemotherapy takes precedence. And when offered, patients almost always accept the chemotherapy. So the unspoken understanding is that I will wait until the oncology recommendations are clear before initiating a larger discussion about goals of care, which might include hospice. Occasionally I simply cannot stay silent and I do suggest that patients question the oncology team further about the benefits and burdens of chemotherapy given their particular condition. I may even introduce hospice as a potential alternative. But it feels as if I am going against the etiquette I have learned as a consultant. Yet how can I expect my patients to make informed decisions if they don't have all of the information?

And when I am caring for a critically ill patient in the ICU, I often feel compelled to request consultations from a variety of those specialists—the infectious disease team to help me choose the most powerful antibiotics, the gastroenterologists to investigate the source of bleeding in the intestines, the cardiologist to determine whether a patient's flagging heart can be snapped back into action. The system asserts that we have done our jobs by having the most experienced organ masters opine on our patient's condition. And they almost always recommend more treatment. And so when the treatments are all applied and the specialists begin to recede, I am often left with an increasingly sick patient facing a full-court press. And there is nothing left to do but to funnel the patient onto the end-of-life conveyor belt, to keep her lungs inflating and to prop up her flagging blood pressure until her body dies.

But that was what the patient wanted, right?

Wrong. Data show that the more patients actually know, the less they want of our treatments at the end of life. A study of 230 surrogate decision makers for patients on breathing machines demonstrated that the better the quality of clinician–family communication, the less life support was elected. Another study showed that people were less likely to want CPR after they learned what it actually entailed. Most people dramatically overestimate the likelihood of survival after CPR. When they learn the real numbers, they are less likely to want it by about 50 percent. In short, when people have a more robust understanding of the benefits and burdens of the treatment they are actually getting, they want less of it.

I HAVE COME TO SEE that as patients become sicker, they paradoxically find themselves alone. They have been shuttled along the end-of-life conveyor belt into a cold ICU with more doctors but fewer human connections. Rarely is anyone talking; everyone is covered by masks and gowns and frantically doing something. In this system, patients are emotionally abandoned in their darkest moments by the same people they went to for help.

In March 2015, a hastily snapped, blurry photo of an emergency room physician went viral. He was doubled over in an ambulance bay, holding on to a wall for support, grieving the patient who had just died under his care. The lay public demonstrated profound interest and appreciation for this unknown doctor. Why? I would posit that Americans are longing for this kind of connection with their doctors. I believe this image touched a similar chord to that of Norman Rockwell's images of doctors in the *Saturday Evening Post.* We all want a doctor who truly cares.

Once it is undeniable that death is inevitable and imminent, the ultimate abandonment may occur. As tension and frustration begin to bubble up from the patient and family—who might be starting to feel that they have been misled—we begin to take our leave of them. Rather than confront our own discomfort or sense of failure, we move on to the next patient. "They're a difficult family. They want everything done." Phrases like this are often heard as patients begin to die on their machines, their families baffled as to how this is happening when it seemed there were still options to try. We physicians become numb to those we came to help.

Linda

Linda and John were at one of the most reputable hospitals for cardiac disorders in the country. Over many months, Linda had become increasingly debilitated by a poorly functioning heart valve. Her local cardiologist had recommended surgery by the "A team" in this hospital. Three months after the surgery, she remained in the ICU attached to machines.

John, a civil engineer, had made advocating for his wife a second vocation. He had achieved an impressive understanding of the physiology of the heart and the treatment approaches to her disease, and spent most of his days drilling the physicians about each detail as it arose. Their interactions were almost entirely about physiology, lab values, and medication dosages. That is why after three grueling months, with one life-threatening complication after another, John had no idea that his wife was dying.

A mutual friend had shared the highly detailed digital journal John had been keeping of his wife's medical condition for the last six months. By the time I spoke with him, he was frustrated and exhausted. Although it was immediately clear to me, based on her constellation of medical problems, that his wife would die soon, I realized he hadn't heard that information from any of her physicians. I gave him my opinion as gently as I could, and he was less surprised than I expected. At my suggestion, he requested a palliative care consultation. Their recommendations confirmed my sense that continued treatment was causing suffering without ultimate benefit to Linda. John decided that it was time to disconnect the machines keeping Linda alive and she died shortly thereafter. John was left with tremendous confusion and a grief that would take years to unravel.

While John attempted to learn about every medical treatment proposed, he had been distracted from his wife's impending death by the din of continued treatment. The doctors, who continued to shoot for cure rather than care, no doubt wanted to do their best for Linda, and for John. But they too were on the conveyor belt—unable to lift their heads out of the chart to look at this suffering husband and tell him what he desperately needed to know. And what they must have known.

Over the years, I have come across many family members like John. Incredibly committed and knowledgeable. They roll up their sleeves and get to work, but without honest guidance from doctors, their energy can be diverted from where it is most needed. Such guidance requires medical experience, which most doctors have, but, more important, a rarer yet crucial skill—the ability to break bad news and reassess goals of care. John and Linda's doctors, expert in the care of individual organs, did not have the skills to provide this key context and perspective. At the moment, palliative care is the locus for this skill set, although I hope that one day every doctor will possess it.

A New Kind of Movement

As patients gained increasing access to high-technology health care, a countermovement was being birthed. This movement advocated for a very different kind of right: the right to refuse treatment.

In 1975, Karen Ann Quinlan entered a persistent vegetative state at the age of twenty-one. Her body was sustained for a year on full life support in a hospital in New Jersey. Her parents, devout Catholics, believed that she would not have wanted to be kept alive on life support in her hopeless condition. But the state felt that protecting its citizens meant requiring that life be maximally supported, even against the wishes of surrogate decision makers. In fact, the Morris County prosecutor threatened to bring homicide charges against her parents and the hospital if life support was stopped. Eventually, after a prolonged battle in court, requiring an appeal to the Supreme Court of New Jersey, Ms. Quinlan's parents won the right to take their daughter off life support. She went on to live for another decade, receiving artificial nutrition and hydration by a permanent feeding tube, until she died from pneumonia in 1985.

This was the first case on record supporting the right to refuse life-sustaining treatments. It has been referenced widely as a turning point in the conversation, which began to honor other options besides prolonging life at all costs. Some began to see that there were more nuanced, and less technological, approaches to health care. It was the seed of a new movement, which has continued to grow, albeit slowly, to this day.

Are You on or off the Boat?

A few years ago, at a family get-together, I sat across from Terry, a retired hospice social worker. We compared notes on our varied experiences with end-of-life care in this country. And then she told me a chilling story.

A year earlier, Terry had been thinking a lot about death. Although still spry, she had no close family living nearby and worried that if she were no longer able to speak for herself, she might be "hijacked," as she put it, into a bad death. She was no stranger to the overuse of technology in dying patients. There was no doubt in her mind that she would never want to be kept alive on machines if she didn't have a chance of returning to her life as a fully functioning individual. She had documented her preference on an Advance Directive, checking the box that stated:

I do not want my life to be prolonged if (1) I have an incurable and irreversible condition that will result in my death within a relatively short time, (2) I become unconscious and, to a reasonable degree of medical certainty, I will not regain consciousness, or (3) the likely risks and burdens of treatment would outweigh the expected benefits.

Then she had informed all of her close friends of this decision. But the best-laid schemes of mice and men go often askew. It wasn't long after she filled out her form that she was taken to the hospital with crushing chest pain. Given how much this mattered to her, she had mentally rehearsed this moment and maintained the presence of mind to bring her Advance Directive to the hospital. But when she handed it to the cardiologist in the ER and said clearly, "I want to be DNR," he looked at her as if she was crazy.

"You can't be DNR if you want us to fix the problem," he told her. She was having a heart attack, he said, and the only chance of curing it would be with a catheterization procedure, during which he would dilate any blockage he found in her coronary arteries. But they had to hurry, he admonished, because they were approaching the ninety-minute window for this procedure. Time is muscle, and every minute of delay could cost her.

Things might go wrong during the surgery, he explained, and if she was DNR he couldn't try to fix them. A puncture of the catheter through the arterial wall, a dangerous arrhythmia that could stop her heart from pumping blood effectively, a stroke, a heart attack. He might even decide during the procedure that the blockages were too dangerous to dilate with a balloon and that she should go for open-heart surgery. He needed the flexibility to treat each of those conditions fully, and her DNR would be an impediment.

Time is ticking, he said. Did she want to receive this potentially life-saving procedure? The risks were very small.

She didn't want to be on a breathing machine, she insisted. No matter what. She had seen it so many times and it had never turned out well, in her opinion. "Can't you do the procedure, but let me die if things go badly?"

The answer was a simple no. "I can't let you die on the table," he said. The doctor told her that if she wasn't interested in the procedure, he would call the emergency room doctors in to provide medicines to treat her heart attack. But it would not fix the problem like he could. Then he made as if to leave.

She stopped him. "Just do it," she said. And with that, she was whisked away to the cath lab, her "door to balloon time" under the requisite ninety minutes. The procedure went well, she didn't require a breathing machine, and she left the hospital after the weekend. But she couldn't shake the terror of having had no voice, no choice. She felt abandoned by the system she had come to for help.

This binary approach to care is often practiced by subspecialists such as cardiologists and surgeons. "If you don't want to go with me all the way, you can't go with me at all," is the sentiment. It's an on–off switch. If surgery is agreed to, a DNR order or a palliative care consultation is almost always off limits. On the other hand, if a person elects or is assigned DNR status, as with Mrs. Z, more aggressive diagnostic or therapeutic approaches are usually taken off the table, even if they might mitigate the patient's symptoms or allow her to live longer.

So what would have happened if things had not gone as well as they did? What if, despite the doctor's attempts to reverse a bad outcome, she landed in the ICU on the machines that she desperately sought to avoid? When would her Advance Directive be reactivated and the machines removed? Would that ever have happened?

You may be wondering why Terry's cardiologist was so unwilling to honor her stated and notarized wishes. I don't know his motives but speculate that they might involve what is commonly known as the "thirty-day mortality statistic." This system ranks doctors by the percentage of their patients who die by day thirty following a surgical procedure. The statistic is widely used by payers such as Medicare and state health agencies, with the aim of providing transparency to patients about the performance of hospitals and physicians against the state or national average.

In theory, health care consumers will choose physicians or hospitals with the lowest mortality rates for the procedure they are considering.

But the problem is that this statistic, with its impact on the reputations and careers of individual physicians and their departments, may be a disincentive for doctors to provide patient-centered care. There have been worrying reports of surgical patients dying slowly for weeks after their surgeries, for whom a palliative care consultation was delayed until day thirty-one post-op. How often are physicians making treatment decisions that put their own reputations above their patients' needs?

Plugging In

The initial attachment to a breathing machine often happens in frenzied moments. A person arrives in the emergency room unable to breathe, or a patient on the hospital ward unexpectedly goes into respiratory distress. And so a temporary breathing tube is inserted through the mouth into the lungs—an appropriate response. Without knowledge of a patient and his preferences, it is right to err on the side of prolonging life.

But this lifesaving action sets a path from which deviation is almost impossible. And for those nearing the ends of their lives, this moment may signal the first stop on the end-of-life conveyor belt. Death has been averted; we have succeeded in this most fundamental metric. And thus to consider detaching the patient from the machine at this point can seem almost sacrilegious. In this way, the patient is led inexorably toward the two-week trach and PEG mark.

Two weeks marks the preferred expiration date for the temporary breathing tube. After two weeks, the pressurized balloon stabilizing the tube in the trachea risks causing irreparable damage to the fragile tissues of the airway. And this is why, if a patient remains unable to breathe on her own at this point, a trach is often inserted by the surgeons to create a more permanent and stable connection between patient and machine. Usually performed in an operating room, the procedure involves making an incision at the Adam's apple, through which the trach tube is inserted directly into the airway, bypassing the mouth and throat. It is held in place by a strap that encircles the patient's neck. Like the temporary breathing tube, the trach is connected to a breathing machine. But it is a more secure and more comfortable connection; the patient's mouth is no longer occupied by a plastic tube, allowing for better oral care, and possibly, down the line, food by mouth. And while the patient is in surgery, the PEG, or feeding tube, is often sewn into the stomach as well, replacing the temporary feeding tube. Unfortunately, in many cases these surgically placed PEG and trach tubes become permanent appendages, connections only severed after death.

Any serious medical intervention should be preceded by careful consideration of the patient's condition, values, and preferences. Some actions beg more reflex than thought—like lowering dangerously high blood pressure or intubating an unknown patient in respiratory distress. But the two-week trach and PEG decision should be anything but reflexive; the potential consequences are so great that I believe anyone being considered for these surgeries should have a lengthy conversation with their doctor—and possibly a palliative care consultant—to explore these surgeries, instead of the usual consent-form transaction. More safety, more comfort, and more life seem, on the surface, to be no-brainers. But dig a little deeper, and there's a serious catch. Patients on life-support machinery often require arm restraints so that they don't pull at the tubes and catheters. They become prone to recurrent infections in their lungs, bladders, kidneys, and skin, due to the many plastic tubes inserted in various locations that shuttle bacteria into places where they shouldn't be.

And by the time a dying body is settled into this new state, it can be extremely difficult to imagine extricating it, for doctors, patients, and families alike. Which is why it's almost never done. Resources have been committed, both emotional and material, risks have been taken by the patient, operating rooms booked, and tissue cut and sewn. Once these surgical procedures have been performed, the risks met and surmounted, undoing this surgery can seem absurd to the medical team. After the hefty success of keeping the patient alive, of establishing symbiosis with our machines, how could we rip away the cord? And for families, undoing a surgery that succeeded in its intent—to keep their loved one alive—can seem an insurmountable obstacle. Why is this? I speculate that in part this is due to the family having played a key role in this intervention—unlike the initial emergency intubation, which usually doesn't involve active permission. The family has let the doctors alter their loved one's body: cut into it, implant a foreign object. And perhaps because they have little other choice, the family will believe in the power of this tube.

Thus these tubes, once inserted into dying patients, tend to remain in place until death. And this requires that the patients remain in a facility with skilled personnel to manage their breathing machines—ICUs, long-term care facilities, or nursing homes. It's almost impossible to die at home once you're plugged in. And this is not the only risk. There are others, also potentially devastating. The risk of never tasting food again. The risk of not being able to take care of your own personal hygiene. Of not being able to turn off the game show that the nurse is watching in your room. Of losing your dignity. And of a lonely death in a facility across town from your family.

For these reasons, the two-week trach and PEG mark is a crucial decision point. Yet it is too often not acknowledged or discussed, done without reflection as a next step in the protocol. Consent forms are always signed, the surgical risks always explained. But the more fundamental risks are not discussed. On the doctor's end, these are difficult conversations to have, especially given our dearth of training in breaking bad news. And we almost never get faulted by colleagues or sued by patients or families for requesting the surgeons to attach the PEG and trach. It makes physiological sense and suggests a desire to keep the patient alive. For some, the possibility of living permanently connected to a breathing machine is an acceptable risk. But there are many who will see this outcome as a nightmare, and to them we doctors owe a frank discussion.

The Big Three

I once took care of a dying patient with Stevens-Johnson syndrome, a disorder in which skin can slough off, causing a burn-like condition. She was bleeding for weeks from her lesions and required daily blood transfusions. With her body days from death, the team met with the son to counsel against performing cardiopulmonary resuscitation when her heart finally stopped. It would be horrible, they said, to put her through this aggressive and futile attempt to bring her back to life. And it simply wouldn't work. But the son insisted. "Do it," he told the attending, "or I'll sue you." Although the attending brought the case to the ethics committee, the patient died before a decision was made. She was subjected to a bloody code in her final moments on earth, administered by the same horrified doctors who had tried to spare her.

There are certain treatments that Americans have come to see as their rights, whether or not the physician deems them to be beneficial in a particular case. I call these "the Big Three," and they are the use of breathing machines, feeding tubes, and cardiac resuscitation with electric shocks and chest compressions. Dialysis is a potential fourth, depending on the family's familiarity with its use in kidney failure. Most physicians feel they are powerless to withhold these treatments if the patient or family insists on their use. They not only are viewed as rights but have also become the de facto rites expected before death.

It seems my colleagues in other subspecialties are more immune to this pressure to perform interventions they deem inappropriate. No family can force a cardiologist to insert a defibrillator into a patient with poor neurologic prognosis in order to keep his heart beating. My neurosurgery colleagues frequently decline to operate on patients with active head bleeds if they don't believe surgery will help—even if the continued bleeding will result in the patient's death. Surgeons of all stripes are understood to have the right to take surgery off the table if they do not think it will be of benefit to the patient. But we intensivists do not have the right to refuse to connect a patient to life support if her family insists on it.

I am not sure why this is the case, but I believe it derives from two main factors. First, no one wants to feel directly responsible for a death, even if the patient is clearly dying. Breathing is binary. Either you are inhaling enough to stay alive or you're not. In which case you die. It's relatively quick. It's very transparent. And so if mechanical breathing support is withheld or withdrawn, the doctor involved in that decision might wrongly be perceived as causing the patient's death. Understandably, many family members share this aversion. I cannot count the number of times I've heard family members say: "I don't want to be the one who pulls the plug"—even in cases in which it is established that the patient would never have wanted to be kept alive on machines. It takes a certain amount of bravery, moral conviction, and strength of character to be willing to step up and make that suggestion or, in the case of a family member, that final decision. It is a lot to live with, for doctor and family alike—and especially so in the face of even one dissenter.

The other key factor here is popular knowledge. Laypeople understand something about breathing machines. And feeding tubes. Everyone knows that bodies can't survive without nutrition and ventilation. And almost everyone has seen a Code Blue on television shows like *ER*, where electric shocks and chest compressions almost always succeed in bringing a patient back to life—in utter defiance of the actual data. CPR is often of no real benefit for many of the patients upon whom we use it, and feeding tubes can actually be harmful for many. Pumping artificial nutrition into the stomach of a dying person increases both the risk and consequences of aspirating foreign liquid into the lungs.

But these facts are widely unknown, even by some of the physicians who administer these procedures. So how could the lay public be expected to know, particularly when these treatments are offered automatically? A bioethicist colleague refers to this perception of the intrinsic worth of these often-harmful interventions as "historical artifact," where the perception of worth that accompanied their development is immune to the developing body of literature that debunks them.

Most people don't know much about the defibrillators that get sewn around hearts. They don't know to ask for a removal of the skull if there is continued bleeding in the brain. Yet when it comes to the Big Three, what they do know might hurt them.

Charles was a thirty-nine-year-old man with morbid obesity. The youngest of a large clan of siblings, he was the beloved baby of the family. Weighing around 800 pounds, he hadn't been out of bed for at least a year. His weight had increased over many years in a vicious cycle brought about by a combination of factors, including a handicap from a gunshot wound, depression, and poor eating habits.

Morbid obesity causes a whole host of physiological problems. It usually starts with compression of the trachea, especially during sleep, which causes a domino effect of organ dysfunction.

By the time Charles made it to my ICU in New Jersey, his body was shutting down. His heart was barely pumping, backing fluid up into his legs, which had chronic ulcers oozing through bandages. He was almost completely bed bound by his chronic illness and had spent the previous year mostly in the hospital, punctuated by periods at home. The admitting diagnoses had become increasingly serious. Where earlier admissions for breathing problems or low blood pressure had required only a few days in the ICU, more recent ones had been longer, some requiring breathing machines. And the most recent admission had been for septic shock. The source was a mystery, and it would remain that way, because he was too large to fit into the CT scanner. And by that point he was too unstable to be transported to the nearby zoo's CT scanner, which was where we scanned our morbidly obese patients. Although IV antibiotics and fluids had initially improved his condition somewhat, he still required blood pressure support from powerful drips. Something ominous was brewing.

The day before I took over the service, he had begun to bleed from his intestinal tract. The source of the bleeding was not clear. Again, a CT scan of his abdomen might have helped, this time to localize any area of dead bowel. But he was even more seriously ill now for transport—"maxed out" on three blood pressure support drips to prop up his dangerously low blood pressure. His heart was beginning to exhibit erratic behavior that foretold cardiac arrest. In addition, his kidneys had failed, so he was on dialysis; and his liver, which supports blood clotting and thus might slow the bleed, was floundering from the high pressures backing up from his heart.

When my team first presented the facts to me, I knew this was not going to go well. I had been told that any surgery to identify and stop the bleeding was off the table—the surgeons wouldn't operate on his abdomen without a CT scan, particularly given that he was so medically unstable. It was a catch-22 but made good sense to me. And untreatable hemorrhage atop profound multisystem organ failure, in my experience, can mean only one thing: death.

I told my team that I thought the prognosis was grim. There were some nods. When I asked them if they thought the patient knew that, there was silence. "We've talked to him and his family, but they just kept saying they want us to do everything," volunteered my resident quietly. I told them that it was unlikely that the aggressive measures we typically take when a heart stops would be of help to him, given his devastating and untreatable condition. Moreover, although he did not yet have a breathing tube, he was now requiring a full-time BiPAP mask, and soon even that would be inadequate. What was the plan for when the BiPAP was no longer enough? Would we intubate?

"Let's talk to him," I said.

I recognized him when I walked into the room. I had cared for him on one of his prior admissions several months earlier. His previously smiling face was distorted by anxiety beneath the tight-fitting oxygen mask. I moved to his side, my paper gown rustling along the bed. Laying my gloved hand on his shoulder, I said hello. A flash of recognition crossed his face.

"Do you remember me, Charles?" I asked. He nodded slightly. "I took care of you a few months ago." I waited a few moments, and then told him I was so sad to see him this sick. And that I was worried because things didn't seem to be turning around. "The doctors have done everything they can to get you better, but you seem to be getting worse."

"But I don't want to die," he said, his eyes widening above his mask.

"I don't want you to die either," I said. I waited a few beats. "But I believe that is what is starting to happen. So I want to talk to you about how we should go forward."

"Please," he said again, desperate under his mask. "I just don't want to die."

As I stood in his room, my residents behind me, I was gripped by a sense of complete impotence. I couldn't fix this. A young man, beloved by so many, so desperate to live, and I couldn't save him, despite my many high-tech tools, my understanding of physiology, and my will. And I had to stand there, with residents and medical students who had come to the ICU to learn the magic of these tools, and admit that they were useless here.

I took a breath and plunged in. I told him that it pained me to be telling him this news but that I believed it was time to acknowledge that death was coming. I asked him what was most important to him right now—to be with family, to be comfortable, to see his kids? But he wouldn't engage with that. He just kept repeating, "Keep me alive, I want to live, come on, doc. I know you can."

This directive, *I want you to do everything, doc,* often ends the conversation between doctors and desperate ICU patients. We've got a lot of *everything* to offer, and the patient's words are considered gold. And so many a critical conversation about goals of care ends this way, with doctors feeling they are honoring patient autonomy by adhering to these requests. But patients in the ICU are often scared, even terrified. Especially right after receiving bad news. I don't think that what comes out of their mouths in those moments should necessarily be taken as gospel. When patients push for *doing everything* in the face of no significant medical benefit, we must give them more time, more opportunities to process their shock and emotional distress about death. Often, I have learned, when a patient or family pleads that we *do everything,* they are really asking for us to stay with them, to not abandon them, to keep them comfortable and calm. To treat them with dignity as they pass out of this world. Not always, of course. For some, there is a value to continuing treatments meant to prolong life even if there is no chance for them to work, even if they will induce suffering. But in my experience, that is really quite a small number of people.

And so I tried to paint a picture of how we could stay close and care for him until the very end. But he kept up his mantra. "Please save me, doc. I know you can."

I realized that I had to get more concrete now. He was so sick that his heart might stop tonight. I loathed the idea of causing this man any more emotional distress, but I really needed specific answers from him. His insistent plea to *do everything* would trigger Hail Mary maneuvers that would almost definitely do nothing except harm—the chest compressions that would break ribs, the electric shocks that could burn skin, and the breathing tube that might be difficult to insert through his overcrowded mouth and throat. And was that really what he was looking for? If he were to make it through that ordeal, would he find it acceptable to live a life on machines—for a day, a week, a month? Without his family? Without comfort? Without his independence? He would almost definitely die in the midst of these efforts, his last impressions on this earth a blur of shouts and terror. All that in place of the warm hand of a family member sitting by his bedside in peace and quiet. I wanted to give him the opportunity to opt out of it. The opportunity we all deserve.

But he wouldn't or couldn't engage. For every procedure that I presented, he just said, "Please save me." I reframed my questions in multiple ways.

"Would it be okay for you to live on a breathing machine?"

"Save me, doc."

"I don't think we should do chest compressions if your heart stops."

"Just save my life, doc, I know you can."

He wouldn't give me anything, just clung to the overarching plea for salvation. What did this man want me to do? He was still making his own decisions, and within existing medical culture, this abstention meant that all treatment options were fair game. My residents, as they had been trained, felt we had enough information for a clear treatment plan. "He said he wants everything done," one of them said as we walked out of the room, a touch of anxiety and frustration in her voice. "And the family agrees. I feel comfortable intubating and doing CPR. It's what he wants."

But I wasn't comfortable with it. At least not yet.

I want you to do everything. What do those words really mean? Many doctors take them as a directive to stop at nothing until a certain point during the code, sometimes fifteen minutes, sometimes thirty, sometimes even longer, when the patient remains irrefutably dead despite massive resuscitation with fluids, epinephrine, bicarbonate, pressors, and enough joules of electricity to the chest, theoretically, to "wake the dead."

All this performed in the name of patient autonomy—honoring our patients' wishes—and thus considered the humane thing to do. And even though I felt great concern that this patient was making the wrong choice, that in his panic he was reaching for a fantasy that would cause him more pain, it felt cruel to keep pushing him to opt out. And given that I could not opt out for him, I deferred to my residents, shrugged my shoulders sadly, and moved on to my next patient.

Later in the day, one of my residents approached me. She wondered if we should contact the surgeons again to ask if they would reconsider operating. "He keeps bleeding," she said, "and we can't stop it without surgery." Hemorrhage is like a leaky faucet. It doesn't usually stop on its own. But the risks of opening up this dying man's obese abdomen with no radiologic guidance were simply too great.

"But this patient really wants us to do everything," she said, reminding me. "And it's the only option."

"Besides dying," I said. She had nothing more to say. But her frustration at not being able to fix this was palpable. I understood. I too felt distress. I couldn't fix Charles.

By the next morning he was no longer communicative. Now it was time for the family to step in to become his surrogate decision makers. I met with them in the conference room at the end of the ICU hallway. It was a large family, given his many siblings and their adult children. I rapidly brought everyone up to speed on Charles's continued deterioration and the inevitability of his imminent death. I expressed my concern about his recommendation that we perform CPR on him when his heart stopped, explaining that I was concerned he had asked for that because he didn't know what else to ask for. I presented another approach, which would be to provide all of the care that would help Charles now but none that would hurt him, like CPR. When I finished speaking, there was a shocked silence in the room. The family had been listening, but I realized that they had heard only the first part of my message—that Charles was dying. Pandemonium ensued. A cousin began yelling and cursing at me. "You better code him, you hear? You doctors better just do everything." A brother intervened in my defense. Then others began to step in, climbing over tables, threatening one another and almost coming to blows. I quickly got my residents out of there and called security.

At this point, I stood down. I didn't feel it would be helpful for anyone if I raised the question of DNR again. Charles and his family all seemed to feel the same way about it, even if I thought it misguided. For now, we would plan a full-court-press resuscitation attempt when he died. We were hitching a ride on the end-of-life conveyor belt. And I had been elected to administer it.

Over the next several days that I was on service, I felt like I was passing a hot potato every time I signed out to the nighttime physician. Running a code on this dying man felt, to me, akin to punching him in the face and would probably have had the same utility. But each morning when I took my place on rounds, watching as he continued to worsen, hearing tales of the nighttime arrhythmias, the massive blood transfusions, I felt the familiar pain of being a perpetrator of an awful death. *First, do no harm.* Another part of my Hippocratic oath I would be unable to honor. This time at the insistence of the patient and his family.

And there was no way out that I could see. In the textbooks, a physician is advised to hand off cases to another physician if she feels morally and medically at odds with the plan. But those are textbooks, not reality. My colleagues and I were all at full capacity on our services. And why should I have gotten out of doing something that would likely be equally distressing to someone else?

Then, on the weekend, bright red blood began to exit his nasogastric tube into the suction canister on the wall. Several cups' worth. Although it slowed quickly, he was now hemorrhaging from the top and the bottom of his gastrointestinal tract. More blood transfusions. More infusions of clotting factors. All Band-Aids. Finally, we were told that the lab was running dangerously low on these essential products. As a trauma center, this was not a sustainable situation. The lab would cut us off at a certain point. Using them on a dying patient could not continue. In a sense, as peculiar as it sounds, this news came as a relief. I had been unable to curb the use of the Big Three. Maybe this development would help the family see the light, now that all other paths to cure were closing off, one after the other.

The lab never cut us off. Charles remained a full code until the end. When his heart finally stopped, Charles's rib cage was compressed and his chest wall shocked multiple times with 200 joules of electricity by staff who knew their actions would never help. I suspect he was completely unconscious by that point, but it was impossible to tell. I was not on service at the time, although I had been in many similar situations. And I expect to be in many more.

At this point in our nation's history, the Big Three are sacrosanct—if demanded, or even perceived as such, they are usually delivered. And so because of his repeated pleas to *do everything* and our requisite response to that request, Charles was set up for an ending that might have been worse than death itself.

I met a friend from medical school for dinner last year when I was in his town for a conference. It's always fascinating to catch up on a few decades of life, like a fast-forward of a family video.

Although we were both pulmonologists, we had taken different paths. Where I had always worked in safety-net hospitals, he had mostly been in private practice. As his practice grew, it had started to provide consultation services to long-term acute care facilities (LTACs).

Although I had been transferring machine-supported patients to the ventilator units in LTACs around the country for years, I had never entered one myself. These facilities are usually far from the hospitals that feed them, both in distance and in philosophy. There was no reason for me to visit. I suppose on some level I knew what I'd find, and I didn't want to see. His description of these places was exactly what I'd imagined.

He told me of a factory environment where body after silent body lay in adjacent rooms, machines churning away. He almost never saw family members, and his patients were not usually conscious or communicative. It reminded me of many of the long-term patients in our ICUs, where family visits tapered off as it became clearer that recovery was unlikely. Whether it was simply too painful or too logistically complex to continue the daily visits, bodies can often outlast the abilities of loved ones to stand vigil.

My friend went on to describe his typical patient, an elderly, chronically ill person on life support. Usually unresponsive. It got depressing, he said, to care for patient after patient who would never go home. It was discouraging to repeatedly perform procedures that felt like Band-Aids on bodies that were breaking down.

Many of my own patients, once stabilized and trached, are sent to ventilator units within LTACs after discharge. Although some will eventually become liberated from their breathing machines and even go home, the majority of these patients, especially those with chronic diseases, metastatic cancers, and frailty, will be ventilated until their deaths. Many of them will return to the ICU with acute, often treatable problems—a urinary tract infection, a severely infected pressure ulcer, a ventilator-associated pneumonia. As soon as they are stabilized, they are sent back to the LTAC. Even though they often remain unresponsive and dependent on machines, the stabilization and transfer feels like some sort of success to those of us in the ICU, some improvement. But I don't witness these patients in the custodial care of LTACs, in their mechanized homeostasis with its tedium and muted suffering.

Listening to my friend's description was haunting and moved me to learn more. The data are grim. LTAC annual admissions tripled between 1997 and 2006, rising from 13,000 to more than 40,000. Of those 40,000 patients, 30 percent were partially or fully dependent on intensive interventions like mechanical ventilation. More than 50 percent of patients with chronic ventilator dependence would be dead within a year. It is estimated that as of 2010, there were more than 100,000 chronically ventilated patients in the United States, a number that is expected to continue to rise. But the most disturbing study I saw was a survey of physicians and caregivers predicting the outcomes of 126 patients at the time of tracheostomy placement, the de facto beginning of prolonged mechanical ventilation for many. Family members and caregivers were more likely than the doctors to expect that one year later, the patient would be alive (93 vs. 43 percent), be generally independent (71 vs. 6 percent), and have a good quality of life (83 vs. 4 percent). The stark contrast of these expectations speaks volumes.

I realized that I was complicit in putting these patients on the medical conveyor belt toward their ultimate, sad destination. And yet what other options did I have? In a sense, the entire system is set up to deliver patients into this custodial care. Where else can we house the many patients who have been placed on the end-of-life conveyor belt?

While ventilator facilities are one of the final destinations of the conveyor belt, other types of institutions feed this system. I'm talking about places that are world-class hospitals, offering highly specialized care for individuals with complex illnesses. They serve, whether intentionally or not, to manufacture hope for desperate patients.

Don't get me wrong—these are places of excellence with substantial expertise in many multifaceted conditions. Many patients will benefit from their treatments. But the very existence of these facilities supports the notion that there is always another stop, another thing to try. Their vans pick up hopeful patients at airports who have flown in to find their cure. Many have run out of medical options in their own towns; others decided immediately upon diagnosis to go straight for the most specialized care. They arrive at beautiful buildings with harp music in the lobbies and excellent food in the cafeterias. Subspecialists are summoned, chins are scratched—but as with John and Linda, discussions about simple truths are infrequent.

To my mind, these institutions at the sharp edge of medicine have a critical responsibility to be honest with their patients. Yet as we saw with John and Linda, sometimes it is hardest to find the off button in those places housing the most aggressive "A teams."

Where ventilator facilities in LTACs serve as a means to continue to prolong the lives of plugged-in patients, these hope-filled institutions, in a sense, prime the pump. Both set vulnerable patients up for unrealistic expectations of our medical system: an eleventh-hour cure, a miraculous recovery. There's no single central conspiracy at work here, but if you build it, they will come. The conveyor belt is here. It requires a loading dock and a storage facility.

WE HAVE BUILT IT, and they have come.

Health Care Providers Die Differently

Health care providers, particularly those in the ICU, have a front-row seat to the suffering perpetuated by the use of excessive end-of-life efforts. I have heard more than a few colleagues express concern about the possibility of ending up that way themselves. But only rarely have I seen anyone take action to prevent it.

A few years back I attended a conference called Mindfulness in the ICU. It was run by Mitchell Levy, a well-respected ICU physician and practicing Buddhist. There weren't many physicians in attendance; the room was populated mostly by female nurses. I was moved to be in the presence of so many ICU practitioners seeking a different approach. It felt like a new kind of hope.

During the lunch break, I sat with several ICU nurses. We shared stories about our management of patients, particularly those at the end of life, remarking on the staggering amount of overtreatment we were witness to and telling of our personal moral distress.

At one point, one of the quieter nurses murmured, "They're not going to get me. I've got a tattoo." I did a double take. "Come again?" I asked. In answer, she discreetly pulled her blouse aside to reveal a tattoo on her left chest in flowery cursive that read "No Code." I stared in stunned silence. I'd heard many colleagues threaten to get such a tattoo, but this time someone had actually made good.

The doctors and nurses I know tend to opt out of the types of treatments I often find myself providing to patients like Charles. And other physicians have noticed the same thing. In 2011, Ken Murray, a retired family practitioner in Los Angeles, wrote an opinion piece that went viral. He had noticed that his physician friends died very differently from the way most patients did. It is a daunting thought that those responsible for dying patients are choosing different paths for themselves than for those in their care.

Dr. Murray's piece is personal and anecdotal, but research is beginning to follow. In May 2014, V. J. Periyakoil at Stanford surveyed nearly 1,100 young doctors who were finishing their training in a variety of medical specialties. Nearly nine in ten said they would choose a do-not-resuscitate status near the end of life. Yet studies continue to demonstrate that often we doctors do not even offer this option to our patients. More recently, the *Journal of the American Medical Association* published two different studies investigating the question of how physicians die compared to others. Although the studies demonstrated smaller differences than I would have expected, the differences were there. Physicians were less likely to die in a hospital or other health care facility than was the general population, and doctors received significantly less intensive care before death as well. Physicians, and presumably nurses as well, do indeed die differently from their patients. And so, while we continue to provide "life at all costs" care to others, we become more committed to avoiding that outcome for ourselves.

I share Dr. Murray's concerns. And I believe that many of my colleagues do as well. It is uncomfortable to watch people suffer, especially at one's own hands. We can feel like assembly-line workers, our only dictate to keep the belt moving, without the skills or training to find another way. If we're paying attention, we know that we're often hurting instead of helping, and that contributes to the profound moral distress that is part of our profession.

Where Did Everybody Go?

My friend's eighty-year-old mother died recently. She had Parkinson's disease combined with a breast cancer that had escaped its remission to run rampant through her body. Two months before she died, her oncologist started her back on chemotherapy— "palliative chemotherapy," he told her, administered not for curative purposes but to improve quality of life. This practice for patients with progressive metastatic cancers is coming under scrutiny for not being of benefit and in fact causing harm. And what's more, the symptom-alleviating benefits of hospice are not available to those continuing to treat with chemotherapy, palliative or not.

It was not surprising that the chemotherapy didn't help. Instead, it just seemed to make her sicker. Three weeks before she died, she told the oncologist that she was done. She could not imagine any more chemotherapy. He said okay, and at the request of the family, the patient was enrolled in home hospice.

Two days later, comfortable in her bed at home, hospice nurses in and out of the house, her children flown in and at her bedside, she turned to her son and said, "I don't think my oncologist liked me very much. If he did, wouldn't he have pushed me to keep doing chemotherapy?"

This story struck me as so sad and so illustrative. After years of aggressive treatment, all hands on deck, my friend's mother felt abandoned by the system she had depended on for so many years. Sure, she had the hospice team involved, and her family at her bedside, but where were her doctors? The oncologists, the primary care doctor—these people had accompanied her through the darkest times of her illness, given her hope when she was despairing. Were they her doctors at all? Or were they just her cancer's doctors, there to dispense treatment but lost to her if that treatment no longer applied? And now, when she needed to feel cared for the most, by the people she had grown to trust, they had simply faded away. Passed her on to the final service.

Diane Meier, a palliative care physician at The Mount Sinai Hospital in New York, speaks to the other side of that equation: the doctor who believes that stopping disease-focused treatment is akin to abandonment. She tells of an oncologist with whom she was co-managing a patient with advanced cancer. He was on the verge of initiating chemotherapy into the cerebrospinal fluid to treat very advanced cancer metastases in the brain. But he confided to Dr. Meier that it wouldn't help. He was only offering it because he worried that the patient would feel abandoned if he didn't. Ultimately, the oncologist did the right thing, and the patient went home on hospice. But think of all the patients who are not co-managed by palliative care physicians. I know that many of them receive treatments from physicians who are just trying to show they care. I have done it myself.

And my friend's eighty-year-old mother was herself trapped in the "more is better" framework, unable to trust her own judgment that enough was indeed enough. In fact, she asked her son to make her another appointment with the oncologists to re-address her decision. Maybe, she told him, if she were feeling better, she'd reconsider and try some more chemotherapy. The irony was that the appointment was set for the week after she died. The abandonment that is rife in this system is multifactorial, but the saddest abandonment is when the patient has so internalized the values of *do everything* that she loses her own internal compass and abandons herself.

chapter four

The Illusion Collusion

A FEW YEARS AGO I was called in as the palliative care consultant for a patient who had been shot multiple times in the abdomen. He had been in the ICU for seven months when I met him. "Please, just deal with his pain," the surgeon requested. "It's too tricky to talk about goals of care with him."

We don't get a lot of consultations from surgeons. They tend to have a very tight, almost exclusive relationship with their patients and don't usually seek out external input. Unfortunately, in my experience, many of their sicker patients have difficult end-of-life experiences, often dying attached to machines and in significant pain. Their patients, I believe, often need us the most. Because the consult requests are so rare, and we feel we can be of service to their patients, we strive to honor their requests in whatever way we can.

But in this situation, it was glaringly clear that treating the patient's physical pain was only the tip of the iceberg. This young man with four children had been robbed of his life as he knew it. Now paraplegic, with intestines mangled and permanently destroyed by bullets, he would never absorb enough calories by eating. Artificial nutrition had been administered through an IV for the past seven months, but he'd continued to lose dramatic amounts of weight. This man was starving to death, and there was no way around it. It might take weeks, even months, but the train had left the station.

I asked the surgeon if I could talk to her patient about more than just his pain, about the fact that there was no chance of preventing starvation and eventual death. Sad as it was, he might want to be able to prepare for this reality, make decisions about how he wanted to spend the time he had left.

"No," she said. "You'll make him give up." She was standing in front of the sliding-glass door to his room.

I suggested that this man might want to know the reality of his situation so that he could communicate with his children and start to say good-bye.

"No. I am going to get him through this. I don't need him getting depressed," she said.

It defied logic. "Please," I said.

"I really need to protect my patient from you," she said. And then politely fired me from the case.

I personally never took care of this man again, but Ellen, our palliative care social worker, stayed peripherally involved in the case. The patient lived for several more months, mostly in the ICU, very frail and intermittently on a breathing machine. He was in permanent "contact isolation" until his death, his skin sagging on his bed-bound frame as his fat and muscle reserves were sucked dry. The surgeon on the case moved to another institution and others were hired to take her place. But the direction of care had been solidly set. Full steam ahead.

The day he was to die, his mother required some social work assistance with family leave paperwork. By chance, Ellen was covering for the regular social worker that day. As they stood outside the patient's room, his mother whispered to Ellen, as if afraid of someone hearing, "I think he's near the end." By this point, he had a large blood clot running the entire length of his arm vein, spreading into the great veins of his neck and thorax. It was only a matter of time before it would release into his heart, causing a cardiac arrest. All ICU staff members were expecting it, waiting for it, a crash cart pulled up in front of his room in preparation for the code. But no one was talking.

The social worker could stand it no more. Despite the moratorium on talk about death, she told the mother that her son was near the end.

The mother nodded quietly. Ellen asked her if she wanted to let him die naturally, to remain by his side as he passed away. His mother nodded yes. Ellen stepped out to find the surgeons and tell them of this decision. They were surprised and, of course, relieved that they wouldn't be required to perform compressions on this man after his heart stopped. The doctor wrote the No Code—Allow Natural Death order at 4:15 P.M. The patient died at 5:07 P.M. Fifty-two minutes of honesty in the chart.

The Fantasy of Perpetual Life

One of the oldest Greek myths recounts the story of Eos, the goddess of the dawn, and her human lover, Tithonus. It is a telling example of the dangerous fascination with immortality. According to the Homeric "Hymn to Aphrodite," Eos asked Zeus to grant Tithonus immortality. Zeus agreed, but as Eos walked away, she realized her terrible mistake. She had not requested eternal youth or even health for her lover. Tithonus did live forever, but the hymn describes his fate, worse than any death:

> *When loathsome old age pressed full upon him, and he could not move nor lift his limbs . . . she laid him in a room and put to the shining doors. There he babbles endlessly, and no more has strength at all, such as once he had in his supple limbs.*

This ancient story speaks to the deep human fantasy of perpetual life and the dangers inherent in pursuing it. From ancient Greece to modern Hollywood, evidence of this preoccupation is rife—from fairy tales promising eternal youth and beauty to the rise of cryonics companies, which freeze bodies in the hope that they can be reanimated in a future where all disease, including death, is treatable.

And the rise of life-prolonging medical technology over the past century has tapped seamlessly into that promise. Doctors and the lay public alike quickly grew to assume that the purpose of health care was to prolong life at all costs. To protect the dying from death. But as Zeus's granting of a poorly thought-through request trapped Tithonus, we have allowed our medical technology to entrap the dying.

IT IS TERRIFYING TO CONTEMPLATE one's own extinction. And now we have the tools to enact the fantasy that we can delay death. In an editorial in the *New England Journal of Medicine*, David Casarett discusses the "therapeutic illusion," defined in 1978 as the "unjustified enthusiasm for treatments on the part of both patients and doctors." He writes that this illusion is reinforced by "confirmation bias"—the human tendency to seek only evidence to support that which we already believe to be true.

Despite the grim realities of bodies kept alive beyond their time, we prefer to focus on the promise of hope, however unrealistic. And in a logic that may be distinctly American, we reason that if some treatment is good, more must be better.

On the medical end, this is almost never an issue of intentional neglect or nefarious motives but rather of hardworking doctors doing what they have been trained to do: Treat each new problem as it crops up, nose to the grindstone. And this ongoing intervention implies to the patient and family that there is hope for real improvement. Doctors consistently overestimate how their patients will do—how long they will survive, how well they will recover function. One study published in the *British Medical Journal* in 2000 demonstrated that physicians overestimate their patients' duration of remaining life by 5.3-fold. Another study noted that patients are more likely to learn realistic information about their disease trajectory and prognosis while in their doctor's waiting room than during the actual office encounter.

You cannot plan for a good death if you don't know that you're dying. And so millennia after its telling, the myth of Tithonus has come to life.

MANY YEARS AGO I WORKED with a very talented young intern. One of his patients was a relatively young and previously healthy woman who had come in with a critical illness. By the time we took over the patient's care, she was almost dead, despite multiple hours of aggressive care by many experienced doctors. The acid level in her blood had become so elevated, it was almost inconceivable she was still alive. Her kidneys were failing and her lungs were filled with so much fluid that we could barely oxygenate her. Her blood was so thin it looked like diluted Kool-Aid. She had no blood pressure to speak of. Her heart was barely contracting and would stop, literally dead, at various points in utter exhaustion.

And we revived it each time, shocking her heart back to life six times in twelve hours. We would not be able to save this woman, but everyone was in hyper drive, seething with lifesaving vigor. Because our main goal had been to jack up her blood pressure, no one had discussed putting her on pain or anxiety medications, which might lower it. I decided it was time to regroup.

I pulled my residents aside and told them I thought it was time to switch course. Time to tell the family, panicking in the waiting room, that we had lost the battle. She would only suffer more if we kept up this fight. I picked up a Do Not Resuscitate form. "I'm going to recommend to the family that we not code her next time her heart stops."

The resident who was the lead caretaker for this patient stared at me in shock and dismay. He had been putting his all into keeping this patient alive. He wanted to keep fighting, and I was tying his hands. The resident walked past me and out of the ICU, clearly frustrated.

To him, it felt like giving up, something anathema to the profession. And I understand, because like me so many years earlier, he had bought into the dogma of critical care medical training hook, line, and sinker. He saw continuing the fight as a sign of caring for the patient; he believed in the illusion.

The patient died two days after she came in. No one was surprised.

Too Young to Die . . .

I have seen doctors—myself as well as colleagues from ICU medicine and even palliative care—fight harder to keep particular patients alive. Even if we know it won't work. The patient might be an especially kind person. Or a woman with young children.

Or, as in the case of Mrs. Z, a survivor of the Holocaust. If the patient is mentally alert—as opposed to somnolent, delirious, or demented—it can be more difficult to acknowledge that he is dying. Each of us is prey to certain biases, and even though it may feel like we're demonstrating our care and compassion for these people by pressing on, we may in effect be harming them.

Carla was a twenty-nine-year-old mother of two small children with no time to be sick. She and her immigrant husband had worked around the clock to provide for their family. Putting in too many hours, with too little help, they had scraped by and made themselves a life. But she'd grown increasingly tired over the past month, to the point that she could no longer work. Then came the abdominal pain. And then the ballooning belly, as if she were pregnant, but clearly not so. They'd come seeking help from us and now we stood at the nurse's station looking in horror at her abdominal CT scan.

It was among the worst cases of ovarian cancer I had seen. Strangulated loops of bowel, cancer caking the entire abdominal wall, liters of malignant fluid. She was by this time so debilitated and tired that she hadn't gotten out of bed for a week. Now she lay in her hospital bed, wincing occasionally if her child, lying next to her, moved even slightly.

The biopsy had shown an extremely aggressive form of this type of cancer, one that laughed at chemotherapy and other treatments. I was consulting on the palliative care team and had been called by the hospitalist (the general internist caring for patients on the medical ward) to manage her pain. The oncologists were scheduled to discuss her case in tumor board later that week and consider whether to offer more chemotherapy. Although I felt the usual concern about stepping on toes, I suggested to the hospital medicine team that I begin to introduce the option of hospice treatment to the patient despite the tradition that we not do so until chemotherapy has been taken off the table by the oncologists.

I was surprised by the hospitalist's response. "She's only twenty-nine and she has two small kids—I don't think it's time to bring up hospice." Hearing that from an oncologist, whose professional paradigm places great stock on the benefits of chemotherapy, would have been one thing. But this was the general internist. Someone I expected to have a bit more perspective.

Her youth, her motherhood, and her general amiability pulled at the heartstrings of her doctors. She would go on to receive another round of chemotherapy, the effects of which—nausea and vomiting—prompted a rehospitalization. Only then, profoundly weak and completely bedridden, was she deemed ready to receive information about hospice. My sense is that this patient's options were limited by physicians who themselves were struggling to bear the sad truth that this lovely young mother was indeed dying.

Fear of Being Wrong

In addition to personal affinity, other emotions such as pride or guilt may affect our approach to our patients. Doctors may be more likely to ignore poor prognoses when they have "invested" in patients by performing surgeries, procedures, or transplants on them. Or, if a physician has made a mistake that has contributed to deterioration in a patient's condition, he may feel an obligation to press on even if the patient will never do well. We sometimes use continued treatment as a surrogate for caring or even as a balm for remorse.

But in my opinion, one of the most powerful determinants of physician behavior is the fear of being wrong. There are a small

EXTREME MEASURES

number of cases that will haunt my practice forever, their memories stifling my desire to speak the truth as I see it. These were patients whose prognoses I thought extremely dire but who, against all odds, had rallied and survived. Or at least didn't do as badly as I'd thought they would. And these memories sometimes render me wary of speaking the truth as I see it in similar cases.

I can count these cases on one hand, but I will never forget them.

GEORGE SAECHIN HAD COME FROM the ER to my service after having sustained a dramatic brain bleed. It was of a size and location in the brain where good neurologic outcomes are extremely rare. If a patient is to survive at all, it will be with paralysis of one entire side of the body and usually with profound cognitive deficits.

Forty-five years old and with untreated hypertension, the patient had been found by his wife slumped in their young children's bedroom, the left side of his face slack, his eyes vacant as the kids toddled around him. Nine-one-one was called, and in the emergency room the patient was lined, scanned, and tubed, medical speak for stabilizing an incredibly sick patient. His initial CT was apocalyptic, showing a major blood clot in his head, causing his brain to shift to the other side of the skull and begin to herniate downward into the compartment that houses the brainstem. If this herniation continued, it would almost definitely result in death. By the time I met him, a second CT had just been completed that showed progression of the bleed, another poor prognostic sign for survival and neurologic outcome.

The neurosurgeons hovered around his bedside, inserting a pressure monitor into his skull, making recommendations for mannitol and hyperventilation—treatments that dry out the brain in order to bring down the pressure in the skull—and performing serial neurological exams. There was a lot of head shaking and worried frowning. The attending neurosurgeon and I discussed options. The blood clot had enlarged and was putting pressure on the surviving brain. Surgery to remove this kind of clot has not been shown to improve neurologic performance for patients, although it is sometimes offered if the patient becomes unstable, as ours was, in an attempt to keep him alive.

This bleed was located at the brain's center, like some undersea volcano. The brain at the site of the bleed was critical for motor function on the opposite side of his body, and it was by now seriously damaged by compression and inflammation from the surrounding blood. He would definitely be paralyzed, but at this juncture we couldn't know the extent to which his cognitive faculties were damaged. And a neurosurgeon would have to pass his knife through a lot of healthy brain tissue in order to reach the bleeding area and remove the clot, a risky undertaking in someone already so compromised. The patient had stabilized for now, and the decision was made to hold off on surgery. The risk was just too great. The neurosurgeons left in a group, with instructions for us to rescan him if he deteriorated further.

Now I was left with the patient's wife, mother of their four children, who had been standing in a corner of the room amid all of the activity. She was clearly terrified and overwhelmed, but it appeared she had faith that all of the activity would result in some benefit. Generally, families aren't as worried as I think they should be—as I would be—and how can we blame them? No one has talked to them, and everyone's running around doing something. It looks hopeful. She gave me a nervous smile and waited. I had no idea how much she really knew. Did she understand that her husband's brain was currently smashed up against the left side of his skull, probably never to unfurl again? Could she imagine, presuming he survived, having an invalid for a husband? What if he couldn't hold his children, talk, feed, or wash himself? I asked her what she understood.

"Sounds like they're going to operate if it bleeds again," she said, in a hopeful voice.

"Well," I said, "I think they're worried that operating might not help. That it might do more harm than good."

She was stunned. "But what if he doesn't wake up? What about his mouth? He looks like he had a stroke."

"He did have a stroke," I said gently.

That was a word she knew, and her face blanched. "So shouldn't they do something to fix it?"

Over the next hour I answered all of her questions, including the ones she hadn't thought to ask. I told her about his grim prognosis, that it was very unlikely that he would ever be himself again. That surgically removing a blood clot wouldn't restore lost neurological function. The best-case scenario was that he would be paralyzed on the entire left side of his body. With intensive rehabilitation, he might be able to walk again, but that could not be guaranteed. "Will he be able to ride his Harley?" she asked, looking shocked. I told her that I could not imagine he would. I explained that he might even die. But it was the second scenario, the one where he would remain alive but with profound neurological consequences, that I felt she needed to understand. This would entail him living in an LTAC facility, where bed-breathing machine units cradled their biological counterparts for weeks, months, and even years for those, like her husband, whose body still had life even if his brain didn't.

I continued. "The surgeons are considering taking him to the operating room to try to take out the blood clot. I'm worried that even if they are able to stop the bleed, he may never wake up. I don't want you to think that an operation will necessarily get him back to what he was." Then I asked her what he was like. What were the most important things in his life?

"Being with his kids is everything to him," she said. "He's a very devoted father." She looked at me steadily. "What would you do if this was your husband?"

This was the question I had been dreading. Although my answer might not be right for their family, I explained, I was quite sure I knew what quality of life my husband would believe was worth fighting for, and what compromises he would be willing to live with. Paralysis of an entire side of his body and face? Yes. Requiring support for basic self-care? Yes. But only if he could remain in his home, communicate somewhat, and be largely intellectually intact. Seeing his children, hearing about their days, receiving hugs, doing the crosswords—those would be conditions worth fighting to stay alive for. My husband, an optimist to the core, a man with a powerful life of the mind, and the most loving father I know, would figure out a way to maximize the quality of that new life. But I also felt confident that if his medical needs required him to live in a ventilator facility or strapped to a bed in a nursing home, he would want to be allowed to die. If he could not think, reason, emote, connect, he would not want his life artificially prolonged with machines or operations. I imagined the profound guilt I would live with if my decision to keep him alive ended up trapping him in an existence he would never want.

I summarized these thoughts as best I could and added, "If surgery does prolong George's life, I'm concerned it might not be of a quality he would want."

She nodded her head.

I felt a terrible heaviness leaving her with this, but I had no choice. I had to move on to my next patient. A few hours later, I was called to George's bedside for an acute drop in his heart rate and a further decrease in responsiveness. The neurosurgeons were at the bedside.

"What's going on?" I asked the surgical resident standing in the corner.

"CT scan looks worse. Dr. D's taking him to the OR. He doesn't have a choice."

Choice. I wondered how much room there had been for choice in this decision. Had the surgeons broached the topic of quality of life with his wife or kept the conversation on life and death? Had she agreed to this? She was watching me from the corner of the room. But the gears were already in motion. She had signed the consent paper, and he was on the conveyor belt. I put my arm on her shoulder as he was rushed out of the room.

When I arrived at the ICU the next morning, an ebullient nurse greeted me. "He's giving us the thumbs-up!" she exclaimed.

I was stunned. And thrilled. Even if he was still on the breathing machine, a thumbs-up said more about his potential to rejoin his life, at least cognitively and emotionally, than any formal neurologic exam. Against all odds, the surgery had worked. At least for now.

But on the heels of my excitement came a whirl of conflicting emotions. What if, as a result of our talk, his wife had not consented to the surgery? Would I have been his unwitting killer? Would I have deprived his three children of their father? I dropped into a sea of self-doubt. I could not imagine that I would ever be able to bring up the possibility of withholding an intervention again.

I think of this case as my "Saechin Moment." Every doctor I know has had one—when a patient who clearly seems to be going downhill rallies. And since one can never be 100 percent sure of any outcome except death—and that only after the heart has beaten its final beat—the doctor has further reason to retreat from difficult truths and instead play out her choreographed role in the fantasy of perpetual life.

George went on to stay in a rehabilitation facility. From there, he went home. When I called recently, his wife brought me up to date on the years since his discharge. She didn't remember me specifically. Yes, she said, he is alive, he is home. He does have many of his mental capacities intact. But she wouldn't match my enthusiasm. She told me that he finds walking too difficult. Embarrassing and depressing. He cannot ride his beloved Harley-Davidson. Instead, he spends most of his time watching TV. He has retreated from his friends, once so important to him. He drinks. This man who was once such an involved father now ignores his children unless he is reprimanding them. Their teenage daughter is in foster care because her mother can't control her. "I am a single mother," she told me, "but with another angry child."

"But he is alive," I offered. "His mind works. His children have a father."

There was only silence on the line.

I told her that I felt terrible for their suffering.

"You don't owe us anything," she said, "you saved his life."

I connected her with social services at my hospital in the hope that they could better support this struggling family. But this conversation left me with a sinking heart, and more questions than answers.

Misleading Statistics

In our efforts to attain some certainty in a world where often there is none, we doctors, scientists to the core, turn to numbers and probabilities. But even though statistics might feel like something to grab on to in a cloud of ambiguity, taken out of context, they can be misleading.

Jeremy was a fifty-seven-year-old man with an inherited neurologic disease that was inexorably depleting him of all muscle strength. Over the past decade, he had watched his father and two sisters with the condition die while attached to breathing machines in LTACs. He was several years past the average life expectancy for people with this disease, no doubt due to the loving care and support of his brother Brian, with whom he lived. Jeremy had received his diagnosis ten years earlier and had lived with steady muscle deterioration for years. He presented with many of the end-stage manifestations of this disease—the distended stomach causing aspiration of contents into the lungs, the diabetes, and the heart rhythm abnormalities, which can be fatal.

Jeremy had been admitted to the hospital the week before I first met him. He had been essentially bedridden over the previous month, his brother told me. On the morning of his admission, he couldn't sit up. While undergoing a CT scan in the ER, his heart stopped for unclear reasons. He was intubated, given powerful medications to support his blood pressure, and admitted to the ICU.

Now on a machine to supplement his weak breathing efforts, he was more alert and quite agitated. His repeated attempts to remove the breathing tube were managed with medication for delirium and agitation, and bilateral arm restraints. This is a step we typically take for the patient's own protection. For those unfamiliar with the ICU, this may sound awful, but it is a very dangerous thing for a patient to pull out his breathing tube.

The medical team had done everything they could to prime him for an extubation—searching high and low for any treatable infection, assessing him for water on the lung, and providing the best nutritional supplementation they could. But each day he failed the spontaneous breathing trials, in which the ventilator support is diminished in order to see if the patient can breathe on his own. The trial would be quickly aborted and the machine restarted to continue breathing on his behalf.

After several days of this, the team spoke with the family about moving on to a tracheostomy. The resident expressed hope that this tube would ultimately be removed, or "decannulated," if and when Jeremy got stronger. Her attending had cited an article indicating there was a 20 percent chance of someone in this patient's condition eventually breathing on his own again. The team's hope was that Jeremy would be one of these lucky patients. The family agreed. They were going to fight.

I was in the ICU consulting on a palliative care patient when one of the residents on this case asked me about medications for managing Jeremy's leg cramps. She summarized the case, and we walked in to examine the patient. The hospital bed was slightly inclined, and the patient's neck muscles were so atrophied that he couldn't hold his head straight up—it wobbled on the pillow. His facial muscles were slack, his eyes at half-mast. He'd weakened to the point that I couldn't imagine he'd ever be able to breathe again without permanent mechanical assistance.

We stepped out of the room. "Has anyone spoken to him about potentially being on permanent life support?" I asked the resident. "He's known about this diagnosis for years. I'm wondering if he's expressed feelings about being kept alive on machines?"

"We've tried, but he's been pretty out of it."

Given this man's progressive deterioration and the typical life expectancy for this disease—which he had already significantly exceeded—I would have been amazed if his chances of decannulation were as high as 20 percent. And even if they were, that left an 80 percent chance he would live a life on machines. I wanted to make sure that he, or at least his family, understood that reality before he got trached. "Shall we try again?" I asked.

There were some nods.

At that moment, the ICU attending rushed down the hall toward us. He had seven other patients, two of whom were not doing well. When I asked him if it would be okay to speak with Jeremy, he touched my arm with a look of relief.

"Thanks. It would be great. I'm completely swamped right now. But the family is open to a trach, and hopefully we'll be able to decannulate him soon. The surgeons are consulting later today."

The process was in motion, with all of the right intentions. But the stakes were so high for this man that I was glad for the opportunity to try to talk to him and confirm we were on the right track.

I walked back into the room. His eyes were now closed. "Jeremy?" I asked.

His eyebrows rose a fraction of a millimeter. This man had been a champion swimmer in his youth. Despite his shrinking frame, his legs still held the shape of an athlete's. Now he was so weak, his muscles so flaccid, that his entire face slipped down and he could barely keep his eyes open. But his raised eyebrows showed me he was still somewhat lucid.

"Your breathing isn't doing great right now," I said. "Can you feel that?"

A slight, slack-jawed twitch of a nod.

"Jeremy, we're worried that you're not strong enough to breathe on your own. The doctors are thinking about putting in a trach." I gestured toward my neck. "Would that be okay with you?"

Nothing.

Try as I might, I couldn't connect with him, couldn't get him to follow my line of questioning. He'd have a moment where he'd nod or shake his head to a question, and I'd be encouraged that he was in there, and then he'd fade away again. I wasn't sure if he was too tired, sedated, or emotionally drained to answer—but either way, he wasn't able to participate in this decision at this point. I beckoned to his family to meet with me in our conference room.

Joining me were his two brothers and a daughter who had flown in from Portland that morning. Introductions were somberly made. Then I asked them what they understood.

"Jeremy's still not breathing on his own," his brother Brian said, looking down. "He really hates that tube."

I nodded. "You're right. He's having trouble keeping up with his breathing. He's pretty weak."

"But he looked great at his birthday party last week," said Brian. "I just can't believe that he can't breathe on his own now."

I understood Brian's surprise. Patients can compensate, even unconsciously, for progressive neurological deterioration, particularly when it comes to breathing. As their diaphragm, the most effective gear of the breathing apparatus, begins to weaken, they transition to using smaller muscles around the ribs and in the neck to keep the air flowing in and out. But these muscles don't have much stamina. One small aspiration of food or saliva into the lungs, one extra exertion, and they simply can't keep up with the demands of breathing. Just because Jeremy wasn't on a ventilator a few days earlier didn't mean he had been breathing adequately, I explained to Brian. "I know the doctor talked to you about putting a tracheostomy tube into Jeremy's neck," I said.

Brian nodded his head. "They said it would be a lot more comfortable for him. They can clean out his mouth better, and he might even be able to talk. Or eat."

"That's true," I said. "A trach tube can be more comfortable in some ways than a breathing tube going through the mouth. Especially for people who will require breathing support for a long time. Maybe forever."

"Forever?" He was aghast. "That would not be okay with Jeremy. I was told that this would probably be temporary."

"I wouldn't go as far as probably," I said. It was time to talk about the numbers—to deconstruct the tantalizing 20 percent chance hovering on the horizon. A hopeful family might not want to consider the downside of the equation—the 80 percent chance of permanent dependence on the machine. For some, that would be a reasonable tradeoff; for others, not. Statistics are only statistics. Jeremy was his own person, with his own preferences and values.

Brian went on to tell me that Jeremy had made him promise, on too many occasions to count, that Brian would not allow him to die as their father, sisters, and other relatives had: tethered to a breathing machine in an LTAC. Jeremy had found that thought terrifying.

"He's really mad at me right now," Brian confided. "He won't look at me. I'm feeling very guilty."

It made perfect sense. Brian, desperately trying to do the right thing, had been loath to give up any chance of success, however small, and had defaulted on the promise he had made his brother time and time again. How do you let your beloved brother die when there is a chance that he might live?

I left the family in the conference room to give them more time. After twenty minutes, they emerged. They wanted to try talking to Jeremy again. Both choices felt terribly risky to them. They did not want to lose a chance for him to continue living. But they didn't want to force him to live a life he wouldn't want, either. And they couldn't imagine ever deciding to disconnect Jeremy from the ventilator after putting him through the surgery for a tracheostomy. It would have felt like opening up a wound they would never be able to close. They desperately needed his input here. It was just too much responsibility.

Jeremy had calmed since receiving the medications. As we entered his room, he looked at me expectantly. This was the most alert I had seen him yet, as if he somehow knew how high the stakes were. But he wouldn't look at Brian. I gestured to the corner of his bed and asked if I could sit down. He nodded and moved his leg over the tiniest bit, a welcome gesture if there ever was one.

I took a breath and broached the subject for the second time that day.

"Jeremy, it seems like you're unhappy being on the machine." He nodded his head up and down, slowly but determinedly. "We've been discussing the pros and cons of putting in a trach," I said, pointing to my own throat.

Now he vigorously shook his head from side to side. No.

"Jeremy, are you sure you wouldn't want to take a chance that maybe, in some time, you'll get a little stronger again and maybe get the trach out?"

Again, vigorous shaking of the head.

"Do you realize that there is a good chance you will die after we take this breathing tube out?" I said, pointing toward the fogged-up tube that protruded from his mouth. "It might be today, or in a few days."

He nodded.

Brian stepped forward. He put his hand on his brother's leg. "Jeremy, are you sure?" He nodded again. There was no hesitation. "But Jack isn't here. He would never forgive us if he didn't get a chance to be with you before you died."

Jack was their younger brother, who lived several hours away. Jeremy considered this fact, his chest rising and falling as the ventilator did its work.

"Jeremy, would you be willing to wait until we could get him here?" I asked him. He was looking down at his lap, considering.

Finally, he looked up. He gave the smallest of shrugs and nodded slowly.

Jack and his wife returned to the hospital within a few hours. We extubated Jeremy shortly thereafter. As the tube came out, while the respiratory therapists were suctioning him, positioning him for maximal breathing efficiency, and rolling the ventilator out of the room, Jeremy looked around with a tired smile and gave us all a thumbs-up. He gestured toward his daughter to come close and mouthed, in a barely audible whisper, "Tell everybody to calm down."

To my surprise, he did quite well for the rest of the day. His breathing was weak but steady. As I prepared to go home, I saw him sitting up in his bed, smiling. Jack was standing behind him rubbing his shoulders while Brian, on the other side of the bed, hummed him a song. The next morning, he was still looking good. He spent the day with his family around him. Nurses came in and out of the room, plumping his pillows, smiling at the visitors. There was laughter and food. There were stories and reminiscing. It was almost a celebration. Later that night, a few hours after I had gone home, Jeremy sat up, gasped, and died. It was quick, calm, and natural, and he was surrounded by his family.

Helping our patients make medical decisions is like a moral slalom course—make recommendations and you might trample someone's preferences; hold back and you might not be providing them the guidance they need. And so numbers feel safe to us; we are offering neutral data and information without any bias or suggestion. And where there is less at stake, cold facts can be helpful. For example, a person with stage I prostate cancer who is trying to decide between the treatments of radiation and surgical resection might want to hear data on the overall risks and outcomes of each approach. But numbers alone can't bring to life the realities of dying on machines. A 20 percent chance of recovery, when it comes to life and death, is significant. But an 80 percent chance of prolongation of life on machines must be thoroughly explored in all of its grim reality. It is critical that the patient understands the visuals and the facts—an LTAC, with its isolation, arm restraints, skin breakdown, and all of the other complications that result from a body plugged permanently into a machine.

Most patients and their families couldn't imagine these realities without detailed explanations from their physicians. When we stick to numbers rather than offering context and a detailed depiction of these realities, we perpetuate the fantasy that cure is on the horizon. And we may lead people into terrain they never wanted to explore.

Overpowering Optimism

Samuel Hains was a young man with an old person's disease. It was one thing for his grandmother or his father to take blood pressure medications, but he didn't want to. Years of spotty medication use were followed by months of complete noncompliance. Finally, his middle cerebral artery ruptured from the constant pressure, and he was found by the paramedics in a dense coma. By the time he arrived at our New Jersey emergency room, the blood clot in his head was large enough to push the left side of his brain across to the right. He was whisked to surgery, where much of his skull was removed to decrease the rising pressure inside and to try to protect any surviving brain. Now part of his brain protruded, bandaged, of course, on the pillow next to his head.

By the time I met him, he had been in the ICU for three weeks, his mother constantly at his side. He had moments of mild alertness and would occasionally squeeze his left hand on command, but otherwise he was unresponsive. Usually he slept. After this much time, with some swollen brain still outside of the skull and a dense paralysis of the right side of his body, the best-case scenario was significant physical impairment. The worst was anyone's guess.

On rounds the first day I met him, the resident reported that the mother had requested the patient be made DNR. "We've been holding off on the trach because the mother isn't sure she wants to do it," said the resident, somewhat incredulously. The idea that a patient might have some brain function was, to this young doctor, indication that all engines should be on full blast. And we were already a week past the usual two-week trach point, which tends to make us ICU doctors uncomfortable.

When I went in to introduce myself to the mother later that day, she explained her decision. "I'm afraid that there are some people who can't take adversity, and I think Samuel is one of them," she said. "I have a vision of him going down the street in a wheelchair swigging from a whiskey bottle. If I let you doctors keep doing things to keep him alive, I feel like I'm committing him to a road he won't be able to turn back from." In a bizarre moment of prescience, upon recently visiting a family member on life support in an ICU, Samuel had told his mother that he would never want to live with physical compromise. "Don't you dare keep me alive," he had said.

"I'm terrified that if I agree to the trach he'll be stuck in a ventilator facility forever," she told me quietly. "He would hate me. He wouldn't even be able to end his own life. I am ashamed to admit it but sometimes I wish he had just died."

As a mother myself, I wasn't sure how I would handle the bitter choice she was being forced to make. A mother is not supposed to want her child to die. And yet I understood. The possibility of watching her only son live with an extreme physical handicap, likely cognitive deficits, and the psychosocial impacts of such an injury—especially given his recent admonition—seemed to me almost too much to bear.

The next day I saw the neurologist and his team in the hall outside the patient's room. They had just finished examining him and were discussing their findings with Samuel's mother.

I joined them. "What do you think his prognosis is for a good recovery?" I asked.

The neurologist turned to me. "He's still in there. He squeezed my hand."

I asked him whether he thought the patient would ever be able to do much more than that.

"Anyone's guess at this point," he said, "but all we can really do is wait."

But, I thought, would Samuel even want that? Or would he have preferred to be allowed to die now? With our medicines and machines, we were keeping him alive. And if Samuel's mother did choose, as the neurologists were assuming, to wait and see how he did over the next months or years, there were still many issues to be considered. I steeled myself to ask some hard questions. What should we do if Samuel went into septic shock from a dangerous infection? Would we pull out all the stops to keep his blood pressure up? What if his kidneys failed? Would we start hemodialysis? Would we continue to treat him with a full-court press as each new complication arose? And what was her final decision about the trach, which she had thus far refused?

The mother listened intently, considering each question I asked. But then the neurologist stopped me. "I don't think it's ethical to limit his care at all. I wouldn't be comfortable with that."

I watched the mother's face. I saw shame and discouragement

cross it; she regrouped quickly and began to nod her head to demonstrate her agreement. At the same moment I was experiencing my own discomfort, even shame, for questioning the life-at-all-costs approach.

I also understood where the neurologist was coming from. Many of his patients who had suffered catastrophic brain damage never woke up at all, and if they did, they often couldn't follow commands even minimally, as this patient could. And so from his clinical perspective, this patient was in good shape. As the swelling improved, he might begin to make significant neurologic gains.

But there was another picture to consider. Samuel might never make those gains at all. Or he might die in the meantime. He had been here for three weeks already. Whatever potential recuperation he achieved would take months to years. And that was if nothing else went wrong. Samuel had already been taken back to surgery three times for continued bleeding in his brain. Prolonged stays in ICUs or nursing facilities, especially with an open skull, are a setup for serious infections. And what awaited him on the other side was anybody's guess. Given the severity of his bleed, physical rehabilitation would be highly unlikely to restore him to the life he had told his mother was critically important to him—a life that prioritized independence, style, and social status.

I myself was struggling mightily. A hand squeezed on command might seem unimportant to a layperson, but to us it's gold. If this were my son, I thought, I would not stop pushing for full treatment and life prolongation at this point. But then her son was not my son.

I went off service soon after that, leaving Samuel's mother with her agonizing decisions. But this case stayed with me, reminding me of another type of risk brought on by our drive to cure. When quantity is automatically placed above quality of life, discourse is snuffed out, and the patient becomes the recipient of default treatments that may actually go against his personal wishes, even hold him hostage. Yet even as I write it now, it feels sacrilegious to have questioned the continuation of treatment for this man.

When I came back on service, Samuel had been transferred to a rehabilitation facility. After an extended stay there, he moved home to live with his mother. When I reviewed his case a year later, notes from the outpatient neurosurgery clinic described him as wheelchair bound and unintelligible in his speech. He was completely dependent on his mother and household aides for all activities of daily living, such as eating, maintaining personal hygiene, and transferring from the chair to the bed. But what haunted me was the description of his behavior, recorded in several of the notes, as highly emotional and tearful.

I do not have any answers here, but I do have a lot of questions.

SHAME IS A COMPELLING TEACHER. It has the power to move doctor and family alike away from honesty and into a collusion of optimism. Painful and familiar to the deepest parts of our consciousness, its mere hint can propel us out of the uncomfortable terrain of uncertainty into the familiar safety of well-rehearsed behaviors.

There are many kinds of shame I have learned in this profession. Shame about being wrong or only almost right. Shame about not being able to save a life. Or about failing to rejoice when I do prolong a life I think will be filled with suffering. Shame about questioning the wisdom of our conditioned response to treat; wondering if my residents see me as weak, a doomsayer, a pessimist. Or even worse, as cold and uncaring.

These moments stay with me, hovering at the edge of my consciousness whenever I venture a bad prognosis or leave the safe zone of *do everything* to question and discuss alternative approaches. Shame, although eminently human, can compel us to ignore our humanity.

Scared Out of the Truth

"Watch out," said the ICU nurse, as I prepared to walk toward the conference room to meet with the family of one of my dying patients. "I'd consider taking someone from security with you." She had heard, she told me, that there were some gang members in the family. "There are a lot of pretty angry people waiting for you in there."

The patient had liver cirrhosis from years of hard drinking. He had been in and out of the hospital multiple times over the past year, critically ill for most of them. And now he was dying on my service. We'd pulled out all of the stops, of course, but he kept hemorrhaging from his esophagus and his blood was so thin that it wouldn't clot anymore. On top of that, he was in septic shock. There was no way out. I walked into the room and was hit by the stale smell of alcohol mixed with tobacco and marijuana. There were thirty-eight people in the room, several pacing. There was a hum of anger and I heard someone mutter, "That doctor better fix this quick." Although I willed myself to smile calmly and say hello, I was gripped by fear.

My residents and fellow stood behind me. I hadn't taken the nurse's advice to call security but was wondering if I should have. I moved into the center of the room. Still rehearsing desperately in my head, I hadn't yet settled on my message to them. Would I tell them that he was dying, as I had originally planned to do? Or instead lay out the infinite number of treatment options I could justify pouring into him? The bags of platelets and fresh frozen plasma. The units of blood, now at ten. The dialysis for his failing kidneys. Those options would, I knew, bring them to my side, at least temporarily. Show them that I was doing my absolute best. And it would be a rallying cry for my residents—send us out of the room with a purpose, a plan. I would be speaking a language everyone could understand.

I felt a trickle of sweat run down my back. I was terrified. Not only of the angry crowd in front of me, but of the potential judgments of those standing behind me, who might see me as weak, either because of my giveaway sweating or because I could not save this patient.

But I followed my first instinct. We had tried everything, I said, but now he was actively dying. There was a stunned silence. "Doctor, you better fix him, you hear?" came a voice from the back. I stood my shaky ground, explaining again that there was no chance we could keep him alive. He was very close to death. I talked about our options going forward. I explained that the blood products we had been giving the patient were not helping. I asked them who else needed to come and spend time with the patient. Time was precious now, and fading fast.

To my surprise, the room started to calm. The feeling of panic and desperation abated and the family started to ask questions. Over the next twenty minutes plans were made to inform the remaining family and bring others to visit right away. By the end of our meeting, I was embraced in hugs from several family members. "Thanks for telling it like it is, doc," I was told.

While initially there may be resistance, disappointment, even anger when receiving bad news, in my experience families are almost always ultimately appreciative of having it told straight. And although I often want to run away from the conversation to something more optimistic, I have found that honesty is almost always the best policy. We must have the courage to switch courses, to tell a family when things have taken a turn for the worse. We must be willing to admit that death is possible.

YET IT DOESN'T ALL DEPEND on the physician. As it turns out, patients and families don't make it easy for doctors to be truthful. A study in the *Annals of Internal Medicine* published in 2012 demonstrated that while surrogates clearly accepted optimistic prognoses and understood their implications, they tended to discount or even disagree with pessimistic prognoses from doctors. Family members often take their loved ones out of the statistics if they are negative, citing special characteristics that they believe the prognosticating doctor could not possibly have accounted for: "Dad is a real fighter." "My sister beat death once already and she can do it again."

It is also a simple fact that doctors are better liked by their patients if they stick to good news. A recent study in *JAMA Oncology* described the profound discrepancy between patients' views of physicians who broke optimistic news versus those who broke pessimistic news. In this carefully controlled study, doctors with good news were rated as much more compassionate than those with bad news, even when the news was delivered equally empathetically. And with another optimistic physician always around the corner, it is not surprising that a physician might shy away from bringing bad news to his patient.

But sometimes, even when we do deliver our bad news, it is the patients who mislead themselves.

Uncle Barry

My husband's uncle Barry lived at the leading edge of life. A forward observer in the European theater during World War II, he parachuted repeatedly behind enemy lines to call the bombing coordinates that helped the Allies win the war. He returned a hero, and went on to Harvard Law School and a successful career. His was a life many would envy, filled with family, friends, and success.

Barry's father, an old-time doctor, was venerated as a font of medical knowledge and expertise, never to be questioned. In their family, the doctor's word was sacrosanct, and modern medicine was considered miraculous. Although Barry chose to become a lawyer, his faith in his father's craft was unwavering. For many years, he served as legal counsel for the Bronx County Medical Society. And as he began to approach the end of his life, he transferred his confidence in his father to the profession at large, despite its many drastic changes since the days of his father's practice.

As his health began to deteriorate, he refused to discuss anything relating to the end of life with me, despite having read some of my writing on these issues. My sense was that he was retreating to a childhood trust in medicine and its miracles and didn't want to rock the boat at this frightening time. He would talk freely about being the second man to walk into Dachau, the concentration camp where his people, possibly distant relatives, stood traumatized and starving, but he could not talk about his own eventual death. He just wouldn't go there. And as his health really started to fail, he became even more intransigent, refusing to talk to me or to his adult children about serious medical decisions that were right around the corner.

And so when it came his turn to die, he wouldn't consider anything less than everything, despite active attempts to dissuade him by his adult children and myself. His body was deteriorating and breaking down in spite of all of the increasing treatments. Finally, he had a cardiac arrest and underwent eleven minutes of CPR. After he was stabilized on life support, with medical tests suggesting he would never wake up again, the cardiologists recommended opening the obstructed coronary artery with a stent. These doctors were going on Barry's own instructions to *do everything*, and this was technically the next thing that could be done. But Barry's son Wes was mortified and called his father's long-time primary care physician for guidance and support.

"Look, if that was me, I'd say leave me the hell alone," said the physician. "You can't go down for eleven minutes and still be Barry. But he asked for this. What else can we do?"

In the end, it was up to Wes to finally say enough is enough. With his father in a coma, he was now responsible for making his medical decisions. He realized he had to rescue his father from his own trap. Wes was in an excruciating position. As painful as it was for him, with the support of his family, Wes finally over-rode his father's stated wishes, reinterpreting his words in the context of a reality Barry had not conceived. He struggled might-ily before arriving at what almost everyone—doctors and family members—believed was the right decision for his father. Barry died soon after the tube was removed.

Like Uncle Barry, a patient of mine, Vincent, became trapped by his own words into circumstances he could never have imag-ined. In trying to honor this man's autonomy, we ended up aban-doning him to a nightmare.

A decade ago, as a doctor in the intensive care unit at the Uni-versity of Medicine and Dentistry of New Jersey in Newark, I met Vincent on his ninth stay of the year. He was a "frequent flier," back and forth between the ICU and his nursing home down the street. He would come in dying, we'd plug him into life support, treat his infection, pump up his blood pressure, and send him back to the nursing home. But then he'd deflate like an old tire and be rolled back in by paramedics within days or weeks.

By the time I met him, Vincent was no longer really with us.

The only signs of life occurred during dressing changes and bed turning when, despite extra medication, pain fired up dormant neurons and his blue eyes flared. There were neither family nor friends from Vincent's life to provide guidance for our treatment goals. There was only his advance medical directive, which he had completed ten years and a lifetime earlier at the age of seventy-five. And a handwritten note stapled twice to the form.

As I've mentioned, an Advance Directive is a legally valid form that allows a person to choose the type of medical care he wishes to receive. It goes into effect when he is no longer able to speak for himself. Nursing homes typically highlight Advance Directive completion rates as a point of pride, a metric to indicate that they are concerned about their patients' preferences.

But the Advance Directives that we receive from nursing homes are often cookie-cutter similar. Almost all of them indicate that the patient wants every attempt to prolong life to be pursued. Rarely is a treatment considered unacceptable, regardless of the patient's prognosis. There are neat signatures from two witnesses, usually the admissions clerk and the social worker. Almost never the physician.

And, sadly, that makes sense. Discussing values and preferences in the event of debilitation is complex, time-consuming, and often harrowing. And since nursing homes are paid to care for patients as long as they remain alive, are their employees really the right people to oversee the completion of these forms?

Vincent's directive was typical for that of a patient from a nursing home. But it was the piece of notebook paper double-stapled to it that caught my attention. It had been folded several times, and the center of the paper was slitting open along its most trafficked fold. The words had been written by Vincent himself in blue ballpoint, in a hand that was just beginning to show its age—a little wobbly but steady enough and still clear.

"To any doctor who will take care of me in the future," it read, "I want you to do EVERYTHING in your power to keep me alive AS LONG AS YOU POSSIBLY CAN!"

And so Vincent's own words became his doctors' guide to his medical treatment. His first three ICU admissions had been for septic shock from pneumonias that blossomed from food coughed into his lungs. On that third admission, surgeons had sewn a tube into his stomach through which artificial nutrition could be pumped twenty-four hours a day. It seemed logical: Stop sending food close to his windpipe and divert it directly into his gut. But it made everything worse. A stomach full of artificial nutrition is even more likely to back liquid up into the lungs. And so admissions four through six were for pneumonias from the tube intended to prevent them.

More tubes sprouted: A breathing tube was sewn permanently into his neck, as he had become too weak to support his own breathing. A tube was sewn into his bladder because of his chronic urinary tract infections.

Like Gulliver, he was covered head to toe with tiny creatures, in his case resistant bacteria, so stubborn that they would never be completely eradicated by even the doubling and tripling of our most powerful antibiotics. And when our antibiotic bombs did destroy a given infection, another would almost immediately pop up somewhere else.

The measures taken to minimize the spread of these dangerous bacteria further isolated him from the world of the living. He would never again feel the touch of human skin on his body, just the clammy latex of a disposable glove and the brush of a paper gown.

In our well-meaning attempts to keep our patients alive, we ICU physicians often play whack-a-mole with illness, batting down each problem as it surfaces. All in the name of patient autonomy. And so I would have continued with Vincent, had I not been stopped in my tracks by an image I will never forget.

On that ninth admission, when I took over his care, I was almost unable to complete my physical exam. This man's body was being eaten away to a degree I had never seen. Autodigested while dying. Even with the most attentive nursing care, a flaccid, dying body has pressure points where thin skin eventually breaks down. In bad cases, the tissue breakdown extends into muscle, and in the worst cases, it goes down to the bone. Vincent's shoulder and heel ulcers were severe. But the one that stopped me in my tracks started at the low end of his spine and spread toward his left hip, melting skin and muscle away so that his entire hip socket lay open to the air. Even as a seasoned ICU physician, I gasped the first time I laid eyes on it.

I am sure that Vincent could not have known what he was setting himself up for when he wrote that note. He could never have imagined that, with our fancy treatments, we could keep his body going even while it was trying its hardest to die. And now he was suffering mightily, with all of the grit drained from his body.

And so this case was the first where I began to openly question our blind trust in patient autonomy. I started to doubt whether this patient's decade-old instructions should be our best guide to his medical management. I convened a meeting with the hospital legal counsel, his physician from the nursing home, the ethics team at the hospital, and several other physicians who had cared for him. Everyone filed in to see him in yellow gowns, and there was a stunned silence.

In the end, we did not reverse the direction Vincent had charted for himself. He died the following month during continued deliberations. Maybe following his written instructions was the ethical thing to do. But I am sure that this poor man could not have known that his last days would look as they did. I, an ICU physician, wouldn't have imagined it in my worst nightmare.

I wasn't the only one who would not forget this tragic story. A decade later, upon publishing a piece about this case in *The New York Times*, I received a letter from the lawyer in New Jersey who had served as hospital counsel at that time. Despite my having changed a number of identifying details, she recognized the case and remembered it vividly. After witnessing Vincent's suffering, she had brought his case before the county judge to request withdrawal of life-sustaining treatment, despite his written words. In her letter to me she lamented the fact that "we are still dealing with these issues ten years later." She told me she now serves on a hospital bioethics committee and is involved in educating and offering legal advice about palliative care and end-of-life issues. Even though none of us could know what Vincent would actually have chosen for himself at that time, the case and the questions it raised clearly had a significant impact on us both.

Vincent and Uncle Barry were different in about every way you could imagine. Where one was a homeless alcoholic, the other was a Harvard-educated lawyer. One never had a family, the other had an abundance of close relations. But both of these men died alone in an ICU, tubes in every orifice, confused and in pain. And both of them had, in some way, set this course by their own misguided words.

Whether in the form of Vincent's letter from the grave or Uncle Barry's summoning of the troops before he went down, their instructions were held as immutable truths. And the resulting care plans were conducted on autopilot, closed to input from others—loving family, experienced doctors—who held information these men couldn't have possessed when they originally stated their preferences.

Walter Miller had put together an "A team" to cure his cancer, but it was actually killing him.

On my first day of vacation a few summers ago, I was driving on the Long Island Expressway toward New Jersey with my family when I received a frantic phone call. Given my reputation among friends and family as an expert on death and dying, as well as my poor ability to set limits, I often receive panicked calls on behalf of someone's loved one.

"Jessica, you need to talk to my friend's wife. He's really sick, and she's not sure what to do. Can I patch her into the call? Listen, he's a real fighter. Don't mention death or dying. Talk your ICU talk."

I recognized a familiar trope. "All right, put her on," I said, as I flew by the first in a series of missed exits to New Jersey. For the next ninety minutes my husband held the phone to my ear as I tried to get us to our destination.

Walter was a seventy-year-old man, wealthy and powerful, a pillar of the community. He had been diagnosed with pancreatic cancer six months earlier and was in the throes of an aggressive treatment plan at a highly respected New York hospital. His wife, in a panic, reported to me that he was vomiting, delirious, and moaning in pain. It was Saturday night and his doctor wasn't available, she said. Walter was due for his next round of chemotherapy Monday morning.

I took a deep breath. This man sounded too sick to turn over in bed, let alone take an hour-long car ride to a chemotherapy appointment. I suggested to his wife that she take him to their local emergency room for symptom management. She refused. "Walter wants his 'A team' at Columbia Prez." She made Columbia Presbyterian Hospital sound like the Ritz. "You've heard of Dr. B?"

I hadn't, which made her nervous, and she tossed in a few other names from the elite fighting unit they had assembled. "Well, they're the best, the most aggressive. That's what Walter wants. My son-in-law knows the CEO of MD Anderson and he told us they're the best. If I take him to the ER here, they'll admit him, and then we'll be stuck in New Jersey. We can't get the chemotherapy if he doesn't go into the city."

I asked her if there was a palliative care physician on their team to manage his symptoms, which the American Society of Clinical Oncology recommends as standard protocol for anybody with metastatic cancer and/or a high symptom burden. The brutal treatment regimens demand aggressive pain management, as any "A team" would surely know. "Walter isn't ready for that. He really wants to fight," she said. "Palliative care means you're giving up. Dr. B says we're not there yet."

This man's fate unfolded in front of my eyes. I saw paramedics and emergency rooms, with an eventual admission to an ICU. Like a panicked swimmer fighting to stay above the waves, Walter would muster any remaining strength for more of the treatments he assumed were helping him. When he finally tired, his family would carry on fighting in keeping with his plans. Then he would be put on life support until he died.

Walter was being treated to death. The more I learned of his case, the clearer it became: His cancer was deadly from the beginning, a tangled web of spidery tissue emanating from his pancreas and melting through the surrounding tissue planes. This was not surgically treatable and chemotherapy would more likely be burdensome than helpful. Yet the family had hunkered down with their "A team" in the swankiest hospital in the New York metropolitan area to fight. And they had fought. As Walter continued to deteriorate, he kept asking for more. And there was always more—there always is. More appointments, more chemotherapy, more promises. Ask and ye shall receive.

By this point I had missed my third exit. My husband's arm was numb from holding the phone and the children in the back were cranky and tired. I had been asked to call the next play in a doomed game. And the "A team" was nowhere to be found.

Partly out of sheer exhaustion, I told Walter's wife the simple truth. "Your husband is dying," I said. There was a stunned silence on the other end of the line. I explained that Walter had very little time left. The disease had not responded to Herculean efforts, and it wouldn't start now.

But then I began to tell her of all that we could do that would actually help him. His symptoms, which had been building for weeks, could be tamed, even eliminated. Palliative care teams bat 90 percent at conquering most of the symptoms that accompany life-limiting illnesses such as pain, nausea, vomiting, delirium, and existential angst, to name just a few. The typical "A team," while busy fighting cancer, leaves the patient alone with his severe symptoms. Anything less than curing cancer seems like child's play. But the data show that cancer patients receiving excellent palliative care live on average two months longer than those who continue disease-directed treatments alone.

Now his wife was really confused. I saw that she was in a terrible position: She wanted to honor her husband's wishes to fight but was no longer sure what that meant.

I suggested we speak to Dr. B together. Walter would only qualify for hospice—intensive symptom management at home— if there were no more plans for active treatment of his cancer. Surely Dr. B would release this man and his wife from their suffering. But Walter's wife was terrified that Dr. B would be upset. "He'll feel like we've lost our faith in him," she said, worried. "He might not want to keep working with us." Despite my assurances, she was reluctant to call him.

The next morning, I left my children in the hotel watching television and headed to Walter's house. When I saw the state he was in, I insisted we call Dr. B right away. Walter's wife was in a state of terrible anxiety, so I initiated the call over speakerphone while she paced in the corner of the room. I introduced myself and explained how thankful the family was to him for all that he had done. Then I went on to tell him that things had now deteriorated to the point where it seemed further chemotherapy would be harmful. Did he agree?

Dr. B answered as if in response to a completely different question. "I'd really like to know if his abdominal pain is worsening carcinomatosis or peritonitis," he said. But all I needed from him was a simple yes or no. I tried again. "The family needs to know if you think further chemotherapy is in Walter's future right now. If not, they'll bring in hospice. Tonight."

Now he sounded annoyed. "It's up to them if they want hospice," he said. "Whatever they want." Walter's wife was getting nervous. Her star player was restless; he might leave before the game was over. So I changed course altogether. "If Walter enrolls in hospice and begins to feel better, might he be able to disenroll and come back for more chemotherapy?" But before I finished the question, Dr. B snorted. "That's not going to happen," he said.

I turned to Walter's wife. *There's your answer.*

It's not surprising that the most privileged and powerful can get the largest portion of the Kool-Aid. These are people who have learned to bend reality to their wills, to make good things happen and bad things disappear. They convene the best teams out there and go to war. But because they've assembled such a powerful machine, it's that much harder to stop it from running amok.

That afternoon we created a different kind of "A team" for Walter. A hospital bed was whisked into his bedroom. Two hospice nurses transferred him into it and bathed and medicated him. His eldest son arrived from Colorado to be at his bedside. The vomiting and delirium stopped. The moaning ceased. Walter lived for another three days. He died in his own room, holding his wife's hand as they listened to the opera music he loved.

Walter's drive to win, so rewarding during his life, almost condemned him to a terrible death. He reacted to his diagnosis in character, bent on conquering anything that might come into his path. Would Walter's relentless quest for cure have relaxed into a different set of goals had he been given more clarity by his "A team"? I can't know. But I do know that all of the players in this drama had bought wholesale into the fantasy of perpetual life. And not even the most powerful and wealthy among us can live in a house of cards.

THERE IS AN ENTIRE INFRASTRUCTURE built to support our fantasy of perpetual life. And that structure does not provide for adequate time and space for substantive communication with patients and families. I remember one pulmonary clinic patient, chipper and upbeat but tethered to a portable oxygen machine. It took us five minutes to get from the waiting room to the examination room, me pulling a chair along the hallway behind us so she could take breaks to catch her breath. During one of those breaks she told me of her plans to fly across the country to meet her newest grandchild. Her emphysema was end-stage, I realized as I scanned her chart and pulmonary function tests. Her time was much more limited than she thought. She would go into respiratory failure one day soon and likely be automatically intubated until her death. I needed to talk to her about that critical decision—to intubate or not to intubate. But it was 4 P.M., there were three other patients waiting to see me, and I was eight months pregnant. I asked her to come in again within two weeks, planning to have "the talk" then. But that didn't happen because she ended up intubated in our ICU and ultimately died on the breathing machine.

Even if we do have sufficient time, most of us were never taught how to communicate bad news. In Dr. Atul Gawande's groundbreaking book *Being Mortal,* he describes his own lack of training in this area. He was a surgical resident at the Brigham at the same time I was. This hospital's training programs have long been among the most highly rated, both in internal medicine and in surgery, and yet both of us emerged without critical conversational skills under our belts. Dr. Gawande tells of a moment when he was shadowing Susan Block, a palliative care physician, at the Dana-Farber Cancer Institute. He commented on his lack of skill with these difficult conversations. But Dr. Block encouraged him, saying, "You have to understand . . . A family meeting is a procedure, and it requires no less skill than performing an operation."

And yet this procedure is not one we have been taught to value. We have not been trained in it, and until recently, we have not been paid to implement it. As of January 2016, physicians are finally being compensated for discussing end-of-life preferences with their patients. Yet there are no quality metrics to measure how the physicians are performing at this task. And the $78 Medicare now pays per half hour of conversation offers a striking contrast to the $106 a dermatologist can bill for a biopsy, for example, that takes at most ten minutes and requires almost no conversation.

And we so often end up trying to make these decisions in moments and environments least conducive to good decision making: medical crisis points in the ICU. Yet there, with organs failing or already tethered to machines, decision making is often dominated by emotion and anxiety rather than thoughtful discussion. ICUs are set up around their machines, the central feature being the "utility column," a floor-to-ceiling metal pillar through which electrical supply, suction, oxygen, and compressed air service the various machines connected to the patient during her stay. The technological imperative is so great that asking a patient or family to consider rejecting it can feel like asking a thirsty man not to drink from a goblet of sparkling water.

Yet most of our patients have had chronic or progressive disease for years, conditions that might have been flags for initiating these conversations long before. Given that all emphysema patients are at risk for eventual respiratory failure, why not automatically schedule a series of conversations with them early on in the course of their disease?

As Pat put it so eloquently in her Pat way, it makes no sense to scoop people out of the river when we could go upstream and prevent them from falling in in the first place. The ICU is not the place for these conversations to begin, and yet that is where they are often happening, if they do at all.

IN AN IDEAL WORLD, all medical decisions would result from a process called *shared decision making*. This occurs when a patient with decision-making capacity works closely with her physician to choose the treatment approach that is most in line with her values and preferences. The patient understands her condition, the likely outcomes and prognosis, and the benefits and burdens of the various treatment options. Although this approach is not for everyone—some people want others, such as family members or their doctors, to make decisions in their stead—I believe it is a good goal to aim for. It should be initiated early on in the course of a disease, in a calm environment, with time and space for questions, discussion, and emotions. The physician's job is to provide honesty and a realistic picture of the future, with a range of realistic possibilities extending from the best-case scenario to the worst.

And the patient's resulting decisions should be revisited as time passes and as the patient's condition changes. The evolving choices and goals of care must be communicated to all relevant parties, including all surrogate decision makers and any involved health care professionals. Shared decision making is neither old-style paternalism nor autonomy run amok. I see it as an approach that supports genuine patient autonomy. But it rarely occurs. And thus too many critically important decisions are made for patients without their input, when they are no longer able to voice their preferences.

In those cases we rely on *substituted judgment*, a less-than-ideal decision-making process for less-than-ideal conditions. In this case, a person close to the patient—whose only motivation should be to act in the patient's best interest—makes decisions with the medical team, drawing from intimate knowledge of his loved one's values and preferences. Yet substituted judgment is rarely as good as the real thing. Cultural misunderstandings, language barriers, questionable financial motives, family discord, traumatic relationships—these are some of the multiple obstacles that can occur when others are asked to make life-and-death decisions for a vulnerable patient. I will discuss the most prevalent of these factors in Chapters Five and Six.

TRUE SHARED DECISION MAKING is not happening enough. We have a broken infrastructure, with poor physician training and inadequate time and compensation to support this process. But I believe the roots of the problem lie in our tendency, doctor and patient alike, to avoid difficult conversations and simply hope for the best.

In order to rebuild this broken system, we must begin by facing our fear of personal extinction and the resultant drive to find something, anything, to save us from our own deaths.

chapter five

Where We Come From

H E WAS SIXTY-FIVE, with the most beautiful dreadlocks I'd ever seen. Even though he was strapped into an ICU bed, breathing through a tube that tunneled through his mouth, he looked almost regal. His dreads were arranged gloriously in a silver gray cascade on his pillow. His son sat next to him in the room, the curator of this presentation. He'd been there night and day, holding his father's hand and channeling strength into his failing body. "Come on, man, breathe," he would say with urgency to his father. But each time we had attempted to wean our patient off the breathing machine, he quickly tired out. Now we were approaching the two-week trach decision point.

I spent several hours with them over the next few days. The patient was intermittently awake, and not very communicative through all of the hardware. But despite this, there were occasional winks and friendly hand squeezes. His son told me about him, his family, his friends, his likes and dislikes. It turned out the patient was a real talker and would sit for hours with friends at the local cafe, playing chess, smoking, and drinking coffee. His son told me that he couldn't imagine his father being alone, even for a few hours. I learned that he did not like doctors and hospitals, and missed most of his medical appointments. He had also told his son adamantly that he never wanted "to be cut."

And so this man, who had entered the hospital with what I believed to be his last flare of emphysema, would probably never be able to resume the life he loved. This vibrant, social man, who liked nothing more than sitting at cafes and talking about life, could only continue living if he agreed to trach placement and permanent attachment to a breathing machine. He would probably never go home again. Or talk again. Maybe never eat anything by mouth. He would be alone much of the time in an LTAC, the rhythmic sounds of his breathing machine providing the new soundtrack to his life.

The choice was obvious to the man and his son. There would be no breathing machine, no prolonged stay in a nursing home. The temporary breathing tube would be removed and there would be no "cutting" for a trach. He would probably die that day or maybe the next. In an ideal world, the son said, he would want to bring his father home to die. At this, my patient opened his eyes, nodded, and squeezed his son's hand. I told them that I couldn't guarantee he would ever make it home, but we would do our best. And either way we would be aggressive about keeping him comfortable with excellent nursing and respiratory care, as well as medicines for shortness of breath or anxiety, should they occur. They understood. I sat with them for a few minutes longer, all of us quiet. But I had other patients to see. I rose slowly and touched their shoulders in a silent farewell. Then I moved toward the door.

The son rose. "Doc," he said, "just one more thing. Can we step outside?"

We exited to the hall. He looked sheepish. "I know you're trying to do your best for my dad," he said, "but I need to ask you."

"Of course," I said.

"You sure you're not doing this to save money?"

The question hit me in the gut, and at first I couldn't find my words. I could see it was hard for him to ask. Over the past few days, we'd built a relationship of trust, and now it felt like we were back to ground zero. It seemed that my attempts to help them reach their decision to use less technology had raised the suspicion that I might be trying to deprive them of something helpful. Then I thought of my white skin. I took a deep breath and reminded myself that it wasn't personal; it was instead the residue of generations of neglect and deprivation that African Americans have experienced at the hands of our medical system.

"I'm so sorry you had to ask that question," I said, "but I understand why you did. I feel terrible that that thought would enter your mind right now. It doesn't matter to me what choice you make; it matters most that you do what feels right, and I want to help you do that."

"Thank you," he said, "I just needed to make sure. I trust you, doc."

We took the tube out within the hour. The patient was kept comfortable, although his oxygen level began to drop quickly. He lived until the next day, when, holding his son's hand, he took his last breath. I never saw the son again, but his question still haunts and saddens me these many years later.

Our nation's history makes it almost inevitable that race plays a role in medicine. And once again, those who suffer the most are the racial minorities who have been chronically deprived.

My medical career has primarily been spent in Newark, New Jersey, and Oakland, California, working with underserved populations, largely African American. I am acutely aware of their difficult medical history in our country, which continues to this day—rampant health care disparities, a history of segregation and exclusion from health care, and abuse in the guise of science, as with the Tuskegee syphilis experiments. I am also acutely aware of my white skin, my different speech patterns, and the power dynamic, both real and perceived, in the relationship between a white doctor and a black patient. I am deeply committed to serving this population to the best of my abilities.

Research clearly demonstrates that African Americans tend to die differently from whites, receiving more aggressive treatment without benefit at the end of life and experiencing more uncontrolled symptoms. They are also 40 percent more likely to die in a hospital than their white counterparts and much less likely to enroll in hospice or complete Advance Directives.

In short, our traditionally deprived minority citizens are at the highest risk of overusing our invasive technologies in ways that may bring no benefit and will likely cause significant suffering. They die in more pain, on more machines, and more often away from their homes and loved ones. In almost every other arena, African Americans and other minorities of color have rarely gotten their fair share of the pie. And until relatively recently, this was the case with medicine too. But now, in a sad irony, with open access and autonomy run amok, they are getting more at this late stage of life than their white counterparts. And suffering mightily for it.

There are many explanations for why this might be so. The 2013 Pew Research study on end-of-life preferences demonstrates striking differences between races in attitudes regarding end-of-life decisions. Simply put, African Americans want more treatment than their white counterparts. In response to the question "Should medical staff do everything possible to save a patient's life in all circumstances?" 20 percent of whites responded in the affirmative compared with 52 percent of blacks. Dr. Kimberly Johnson, an African American health care researcher at Duke University who led a session I attended at the American Academy of Hospice and Palliative Medicine (AAHPM) annual assembly, explained it this way in her presentation: "When whites were getting hospice and looking for alternatives in the sixties and seventies, blacks were just trying to get health care." More seems better when compared to nothing. There are other factors too. As we know, less communication translates into worse care. There are many reasons why communication between a white doctor and a black patient, a common pairing, might be suboptimal.

An African American social worker once cautioned me against recommending the withholding of treatments to African American patients. She felt that this could polarize the conversation and erode trust. White doctors may sense this and be relatively quick to end the conversation about withdrawing or withholding treatments if they detect resistance. Or they may avoid bringing it up altogether. As for the patients, they may not trust information coming from a system to which they were long denied access—if they get that information at all. Whatever the reason, effective information transfer is not possible with communication that is broken, aborted, or never attempted in the first place.

Miss Mabel

My patient was an elderly African American woman with a bad heart. She'd been admitted with her fifth episode of fluid on the lungs in eight months, and her breathing had been touch and go for days. Finally, our medicines kicked in, and her sick kidneys began to release liters upon liters of urine, drying out her lungs enough that she was no longer in immediate danger of being intubated. But it was only a matter of time before another flare-up would bring her back to us, and I knew that a conversation about a breathing tube was way overdue.

I entered her room without a lot of time to spare. We were planning to discharge her from the ICU to the hospital floor later that day, and a room was in the process of being cleaned upstairs. The patient acknowledged me nervously and sat up a bit in the bed. Her daughter, usually present at our meetings, wasn't due in until later, but I was afraid to miss the opportunity to have a goals-of-care discussion, which hadn't happened so far.

I pulled up a chair and sat next to her. "I'm so glad you're feeling better," I said. "This must have been scary." She nodded cautiously. Then I dove in. I began to talk about breathing machines. She had been intubated on her third admission, so there was a reference point. I explained that her heart failure was accelerating and that we might not be successful in getting her off the ventilator the next time she got intubated.

"Would you want us to put you on a breathing machine if our medicines couldn't treat your breathing quickly enough?" I asked.

Her face closed up. She was leaning as far away from me as she could, back into the pillows. I couldn't tell if she was angry or perhaps terrified. I asked what she was thinking but got no response. Was there dementia? Was she confused? She simply wouldn't answer.

At that moment, I felt a gentle tap on my arm and turned around to see one of the social work interns, a young African American woman. She must have been standing behind me for a

while. I felt a slight tug of concern. Had I somehow been culturally insensitive?

"Mind if I give it a try?" she asked quietly.

I stood up and gestured to my vacated seat. "Please," I said.

She sat down next to my patient. Picking up her hand, she
smiled at the elderly woman. There was no talking for several
beats. The woman visibly relaxed, then smiled back.

"Miss Mabel," the intern said in an admiring voice, "where
did you get your hair done? It's lovely!"

And they began to talk.

It would never have occurred to me to talk to my patient—
this one or any other—about her hair. It wouldn't have occurred to me to call her Miss Mabel. One might argue that the
patient's hesitation to talk to me had nothing to do with race,
that she closed up because I was hurried and insensitive. But
from then on, I began to notice how Chaplain Betty Clark and
Reverend Donald Miller were addressing elderly African American patients, with a quiet calm and respectful deference that felt
almost Southern in its cadence. I realized that I needed to slow
down and set a different tone—something that has proven challenging for me, with my fast-paced, East Coast urgency. This
was not something I'd ever learned in medical school. I realized
that I'd likely been inadvertently offending my patients for years.
I promised myself I would do everything I could to change my
approach.

We Are Where We Come From

Race, religion, culture, class, and language—these are all socio-
cultural frameworks that shape our preferences in collective ways
and sit at the table alongside patients, families, and doctors as we

struggle through these difficult decisions. There is also another set of variables that can impact end-of-life choices—those more particular to the person or family system. These variables might include the dance of family dynamics, individual personalities, and histories of trauma, to name but a few.

Medical schools try to prepare students for the broad array of patients they will meet. In my day, we had about ten hours of what was called cultural competency training over four years. Ten hours may be a generous estimate; when I asked several doctor friends of my generation how much training they received in their programs, almost all responded with a simple "None." More than twenty years later, I cannot help but chuckle at the implication that I would have achieved any level of competence from my classroom tour of different cultures. Today, many medical schools have changed their teaching goals from cultural competence to cultural humility, which to me seems much more attainable and respectful. This new approach is about asking questions, listening, and learning. And acknowledging that we can never be experts on someone else's life.

But we do have to start somewhere. One framework for cultural context that I have found helpful offers two broad categories: individualist (North America and northern Europe) and collectivist (Asia and southern Europe). Although this simplistic subgrouping belies the complexity of the matter, I have seen evidence of this differentiation frequently and have found the approach helpful at times. Collectivist cultures often prioritize the family's needs over those of the patient, and the decision-making process belongs largely to the family. Individualist culture, which we have already discussed at length, puts the patient at the center of the decision-making process. In a 2000 study comparing attitudes on patient autonomy between physicians in Japan and those in the United States, 80 percent of U.S. physicians agreed that the patient should be told of a diagnosis before the family, while only 17 percent of Japanese physicians agreed. But in a sign that these cultural differences are far from immutable, in 2015, after palliative care had penetrated further into Japan's society, that number rose to 82 percent. Thus, while these collective values or norms can be powerful factors in patients' decisions, they can also shift over time.

In sum, each patient is a constellation of beliefs, history, culture, and other often unknowable variables, and these interact to create complex, and often inconsistent, beings. For the busy clinician or the young trainee, it is sometimes easier to attribute difficult or complicated interactions with patients and families to a "cultural" issue and back off without probing further. But, in my experience, this form of cultural deference can sometimes be dangerous.

Mrs. Rahim

Mrs. Rahim had been rushed to the hospital a month earlier, her intestines obstructed to the point of bursting. After four hours of emergency surgery, she emerged with a colostomy bag taped to her abdomen, the obstruction temporarily bypassed. But the roots of the cancerous fronds that had caused the problem could not be cut out. The surgeon's operative report was a grim litany of the ravages of ovarian cancer, with tumors studding almost every nook and cranny of her abdomen. The omentum, the fatty blanket overlying the abdominal cavity, was "caked" with tumor.

Already debilitated, malnourished, and immunocompromised from months of intestinal obstruction, she went into septic shock after the surgery. Her already compromised kidneys—also being strangled by cancer—stopped working altogether. Then somehow her arm got loose and she pulled out her own breathing tube. Still, she eventually stabilized enough to be transferred out of the ICU onto the step-down unit. But she became increasingly depressed, begging her family to take her back to her native country before she died. As the situation worsened, she let go of that dream. But she stopped eating, telling her nurse she wanted to die. When her family pressured her, she resumed.

I was called in as the palliative care consultant by her surgical team to work with the patient and the family to determine the next steps. The team told me that the patient's family was making the decisions. Even though her family spoke English, the patient did not. Her language isn't common in this country, and although I tried to secure our single interpreter for the meeting, he wasn't available when I was able to see the patient. It is no surprise that patients receive safer and more satisfactory care when they are provided with professional language services. Unfortunately, we may not always be able to access those services when we need them.

On this visit, the patient lay quietly in her bed with her blanket pulled up over her head. The family hovered around her bed, very protective and attentive. She was clearly the matriarch, and they spoke proudly of her fierce independence and strength. Now is not a good time to talk to her, they told me. She needs to be positive and get back her strength. "In our culture," they explained, "people talk to the *family* about serious matters."

It's well known—and it makes good sense—that health outcomes improve when doctors provide culturally sensitive care. On my whirlwind tour of culture during medical school, we touched on China, India, and Africa, learning in broad strokes about each region's beliefs about health care, disease, the afterlife, and communication. We learned about funeral rituals and exotic-sounding practices that might take place in the patient's room. But the takeaway was this: Culture is something to be deferred to. If there is ever any suggestion that a clash of opinion is due to a cultural difference, we doctors should back off immediately, for our patient's sake. If the patient or family insists on certain approaches to care, we should do our best to honor them, even if we disagree.

And so, when Mrs. Rahim's family members told me not to speak directly to her, I accepted their dictum. Without an interpreter, I couldn't even try. But I didn't probe to find out why they felt I should not talk to her. I didn't ask the patient for permission to bypass her and consult her family on decisions. So, with hand gestures and whispers, we decided to meet outside the room to talk.

I explained to her family that she had a very aggressive type of cancer. "But the doctors took it out," her daughter said reassuringly, her hand on my arm. "They told us that they washed out the stomach before they closed her." *Washing.* This is surgery-speak for spritzing sterile saline onto the operative site after a procedure, to clean up the remaining blood and debris. The family had misunderstood. They thought the cancer was out, or at least held at bay.

And so it was my job to break the bad news. The cancer was everywhere, I told them, and it was only a matter of time before it grew another tentacle to obstruct another organ. Thus there was an urgent need to make some decisions. Specifically, would she want to opt out of all of the ICU interventions that were waiting on the sidelines? For this patient, I explained—elderly and sick with metastatic cancer—our electric shocks, chest compressions, breathing machines, and blood pressure support medications would almost surely not bring her back and would likely add suffering. Even more important, it seemed to me she had made it clear that she didn't want this approach by ripping out her breathing tube and saying she wanted to return to her country to die.

"You are right," the American granddaughter said to me, nodding, "this probably isn't what she would want." She told me she would talk to her mother, the patient's eldest daughter and main decision maker, who wasn't with us now. "I will tell you what we decide tomorrow."

I presented my view that it was her grandmother's wishes that were most important here. "What would she want if she knew that she was dying? That there was a risk of dying on machines?"

"We will get back to you," she responded politely.

But there were no decisions made the next day or the following. There were always more people to consult. More elders to weigh in. The son-in-law was named as key to the decision-making process, but he still hadn't made an appearance, despite my requests to speak to him. I continued to meet with the family over the course of a week, waving to the impassive patient as her family gathered their belongings to come meet me in the hallway. I felt increasingly discomfited by her absence in this conversation, and guilty. I was doubly concerned because I didn't seem to be getting through to the family: They didn't appear to understand the shrinking timeline for opting out of ICU treatment. And her medical situation was deteriorating fast.

I decided it was time to get more assertive. I sat down in the room next to the daughter, her mother in the bed beside us with her blanket over her head, and said the words. "Your mother is dying," I said. The daughter stared at me. Then she removed her purse from her lap, laid her head on her knees, braced her hands on the floor, and wept.

Yet no decisions were forthcoming. And now this daughter,

the primary decision maker, began to avoid me. "The patient's daughter has asked that you don't come back to talk to them," the surgical resident told me. "She says it's too much for her. She told me that in her culture, a daughter could get cursed if she makes a decision that would result in her mother's death."

Now I was worried. I huddled outside the patient's room with my team and the interpreter. I told them that I thought it was time to talk to the patient herself. She needed to know, I said, or she would surely end up in a situation she did not seem to want. Didn't she deserve the chance to opt out? But the interpreter shook his head. He said he would be very uncomfortable translating if I were to tell the patient that she was dying. That was not done in their culture, he said.

What was my responsibility here? I had a dying patient who was hurtling toward the ICU, a place that would offer her nothing but maybe a few extra days attached to machines and a cold, metallic death. And I was almost certain she didn't want that. Yet I had, in effect, been handcuffed from talking to her directly. And in a sadly ironic twist, given my disparate roles, I might eventually be her ICU doctor—I might find myself overseeing treatments that I knew would not be of benefit to a woman who I was convinced didn't want them.

When it comes to dying and the risks of a bad death, does our responsibility as doctors override cultural values? Is it ever acceptable to bypass cultural norms and expectations in an attempt to get to the human truth? While in many cultures the tradition is to work through the family rather than talk directly to the patient during the dying process, the potential for harm is great, and patients may unintentionally be held hostage by their families.

Of course, this situation can occur even when culture is not a factor. I've certainly worked with families from backgrounds similar to mine in which a grieving and overwhelmed daughter is unable to process information and focus on her mother's needs. In those situations, however, I would not be held back by considerations of culture, but would press forward and probe. Could I possibly do that here? Is it ever appropriate to override cultural concerns?

There are no easy answers. American medical culture values the physician–patient relationship over the physician–family one. But we also understand the importance of cultural sensitivity. Had I pulled up a chair to the patient's bed despite her family's protests and asked her if she wanted to know more, they probably would have been angry. I would risk losing their trust, which might make things worse for the patient. And even if I did approach the patient, would I actually be able to establish a helpful connection even with a willing interpreter, which I did not have?

And so I didn't try. I walked away from the case despite my concerns, and I must admit I accepted my banishment with some relief.

A few days later, as ICU attending, I walked past room 5 and saw Mrs. Rahim. Her kidneys had finally failed. Although she was still being cared for by the ward team, she received her dialysis in an ICU room where there was more nursing support. Her hands were again tied down to the bed due to her repeated attempts to pull the catheter out of her neck. She lay, resigned, as the machines sucked, cleaned, and replaced her blood. She had shrunk in size since I last saw her. But she seemed more alert, desperate, and scared than she had before. Her eyes caught mine, and she immediately began beckoning me with her hand, despite the fact that it was tied down at the wrist. I didn't know what to do. It was the first time I'd seen her alone. But her hand flapping only grew more urgent, and I decided to go to her. It was the right thing to do, I decided, the human thing to do. I went into her room with a nurse who, fortuitously, spoke her language.

"What is happening?" the patient asked, terror in her eyes.

It took a minute for words to come. "Your family thought it would be better for me to talk to them about your medical condition," I said. "Are you saying that you would like me to talk directly to you?"

She nodded hesitantly.

"Do you understand what is happening? Why you're here?"

"No. I want to go back to my room upstairs and be with my family. I don't like this place." She paused. Then she asked, "Do I have cancer?"

Her family had told me that this had been her biggest fear for years. And it was the information that they had been desperately trying to keep from her. Yet she had asked me directly. I nodded slowly. Then I realized that this was going to be a long meeting and I wanted to be able to sit down next to her and hold her hand. I asked the nurse to tell the patient I was stepping into the hallway to grab a chair. But as I searched the hall for a chair, I saw two of her daughters enter the room. I stood stock-still, feeling as if I had been caught red-handed. There was a quick exchange as they realized that their mother had just received this dreaded news. And then fury. I was three rooms away when I heard them begin to yell at the nurse. "What kind of unethical doctor would tell a scared woman that she is dying?"

I felt paralyzed. Somewhere I knew that I should talk to them, acknowledge their anger, and maybe even apologize. I wanted to take their rage away from this vulnerable patient's bedside. But I was numb. I realized that I didn't know how to fix whatever it was that I had done. And, I reasoned, trying to fix it might make things worse for the patient. I turned and walked out of the ICU.

Although I could somewhat justify it, I felt like a thief sneaking out the back door.

Weeks earlier, when still officially involved, I had referred this case to the ethics committee. They were struggling with it themselves. They were scheduled to meet again soon after this incident. Despite the fact that I was no longer involved, I came to the meeting to offer background and my own perspective. Community members and professionals of many stripes sit on these committees to provide a breadth of experience and knowledge. In addition, that day there were several doctors, nurses, and social workers present who had cared for this family. The room divided rapidly into what felt to me like two camps, without much overlap. On one side were people who felt that the family's stated cultural needs were closest to the truth and should not be questioned. The other camp, consisting largely of the doctors responsible for this patient's care, felt that interpreting this case primarily from the lens of culture might be obscuring other important issues.

In the end, the ethics committee recommended we probe further, in order to understand the cultural context. While aligned with textbook teaching, the recommendation was not helpful for those providing direct care to this patient. It did not address the messy realities, where motives are complex, families are overwhelmed, patients are weak and vulnerable, and the time for action is limited.

Mrs. Rahim died the following week in the ICU while receiving dialysis. She was tied down to the bed and alone in the sterile room. She had been repeatedly transferred back and forth from the step-down unit to the ICU, depending on her blood pressure. The family had continued to refuse to talk about goals of care with the doctors who came after me.

This case has left me with no easy or clear answers. Would it

EXTREME MEASURES

have been better to speak directly to the patient from the start, despite the family's insistence that I stay away from her? Or should I have continued to care for her as best I could within the family's stated cultural proscriptions and hope against all odds that she somehow died peacefully? With my lack of formal training in this realm, I do not claim to know the answers to these questions. In fact, I wonder if there are actual answers, or if, again, there are only more questions.

Is there a point at which we doctors should hold cultural differences as less important than the simple realities of being human? To put a different spin on it, might there be instances where prioritizing cultural needs proves inhumane?

Religion

Roland Dreux was a fifty-eight-year-old Haitian man who presented in respiratory failure. His daughter and her husband had brought him in from their home, where he had been living for two weeks due to his accelerating weakness during the previous year: falls, difficulty getting out of a chair, and, finally, an inability to ascend the stairs to his room. Over the previous days, the daughter told us, he began to have trouble lifting a fork to his mouth, and she had found him occasionally bending his head and eating directly off his plate. Like so many of my patients without health insurance, they had put off coming to the hospital in the hope that he would somehow get better. But by the morning of his admission, he had become unable to breathe deeply, and the rising carbon dioxide levels in his blood were causing somnolence and confusion. In the emergency room he was immediately intubated and put on a breathing machine, which quickly washed the carbon dioxide out of his blood and woke him back up.

When I saw him on rounds the next morning, he was completely alert and responsive to an interpreter. However, he had evidence of chronic muscle wasting, which suggested that this was a progressive and long-standing process, one that was unlikely to improve. He appeared terrified and his eyes were begging for information. We had none yet but proceeded over the next few days to conduct multiple tests and consult our neurologists. Every day that passed there was a new test to be done. And so my interactions with him were all focused on his comfort and our search for a diagnosis—I couldn't bring myself to tell him that I was highly concerned that we wouldn't be able to turn things around.

Over those next two weeks, we came up empty. We had ruled out the more obvious causes of his illness, such as infection or stroke, and the neurologists suspected that Mr. Dreux's disease fell into the category of the progressive neuromuscular disorders. These tend to follow a predictable and linear course of deterioration, and from the looks of it, Mr. Dreux was at the end stage. In order to determine the exact disease within this category, the neurologists would have to do more invasive and painful testing, including muscle biopsies and nerve conduction studies. But achieving a diagnosis didn't mean there were treatments for it. I sat down with the neurologist to ask whether she thought this was reversible, whether he would ever be able to live off machines.

She raised her eyebrows. "Of course not. But we need to have a diagnosis."

I was shocked by her coldness. She was clearly more interested in naming the disease than in the human being on the bed. When I explained that we needed to determine with him whether to continue life support or to consider removing it and managing his symptoms, she looked at me askance.

"If you take these tubes out, he'll die. . . . What is there to talk about?"

"I wouldn't want to live this way," I said, "so I don't feel very good about not offering him the option to refuse life on a machine. He may choose to let nature take its course. Or not. But either way, isn't it his decision?"

The neurologist was still uncomfortable. "I don't want to be a party to euthanasia," she said.

We were approaching the two-week trach decision point and it was time to assess the goals of care. I wanted to present him with an alternative care plan that would include taking the breathing tube out and allowing him to die in the most natural and comfortable way possible.

I arranged a conference at the patient's bedside with his daughter and her husband. I started out by holding the patient's withered hand and, speaking through an interpreter, told him I could only imagine how stressful and scary this was, not knowing what might happen. He nodded and waited to hear more. I reviewed the medical history and information explaining that, although the specific disease was still undetermined, the physicians all agreed that it was an irreversible process. There were other painful and risky tests we could do to better describe or name the disease, but none that would change its outcome. I sat with them for a period of time and explained the various options: have the surgeons place permanent tubes for life support and send him to a nursing home; or remove the temporary life-support tubes and aggressively treat all symptoms, including anxiety, shortness of breath, pain, and thirst. I watched the patient's face carefully as I laid this awful news before him. His expression had gone from terrified yet hopeful to blank. He had stopped nodding or responding. I left the family alone to talk. After twenty minutes of praying together at the bedside, they emerged. "We will go home and think about it," said the daughter.

The daughter and her husband were not at the hospital the next day. Nor the following. My attempts to reach them failed. And Mr. Dreux would not engage at all with the interpreter and lay staring straight up at the ceiling. I didn't have time to sit with him and try to hold his hand. All I could do was tell my team to start him on a medicine for anxiety, which we did.

Several days later, Mr. Dreux remained uncommunicative. He looked so sad that I felt it would be cruel to keep pushing him to talk. It seemed I would have to work with his surrogates, although I had not seen his daughter or son-in-law for days. I reached the daughter at home. She was silent on the other end, not offering any information, any decisions. I suggested that she return to the hospital to spend time with her anxious father. I also said that we were still waiting for their input as to the next steps, as we had reached a serious decision point about the trach. She told me that she would be in on Sunday to "give the final decision." Sunday was two days away and I would not be in the hospital—the shift would be covered by a doctor who was covering multiple wards, not someone who could devote time to discussing these principles. Delaying the conversation would be putting the patient at further risk of tracheal breakdown from the temporary breathing tube. He was already at the two-week mark. I told her that we could not wait until Sunday to discuss it. "I cannot come before then," she said. "I'll be there on Monday." And the phone went dead.

Was it denial? Fear? I couldn't know but I realized that I had no choice but to go back to the patient. It felt unkind to request a decision from him without family support in the room, but I felt I had no choice.

Accompanied by an interpreter, I tried to elicit his thoughts and feelings. This time he tried to respond, but the communication barrier was too great. He was too weak to write, unable to talk with the tube in his mouth, and looked like a deer in the headlights every time I asked him a question. I tried a few more times but found it increasingly hard to face his worried eyes. And so I decided that until we could have this conversation with his daughter, we would keep Mr. Dreux heavily sedated on anxiety medications.

On Monday, the daughter and her husband arrived. I found them standing outside the patient's room waiting to speak to me. The nurse later told me they had not entered the room prior to my arrival. Standing rigidly, clutching her purse, the daughter said she had decided that her father should receive the PEG and trach and be sent to a nursing home.

"I am religious," she said, "and I could never live with myself if I didn't do everything possible to prolong his life. My God tells me I cannot kill my father."

I reminded her that it would be the disease killing him, not she. But her decision was made. She turned and walked out of the ICU with her husband, and I never saw her again. Mr. Dreux was taken to the operating room the next day for tube placements and then sent to a nursing home, where his remaining time would be spent lying face up in a bed, tubes sewn into his neck and stomach until he eventually died.

What informed the daughter's decision? Was it religion or denial? Fear of God or cowardice? This daughter knew her father's values better than I ever could, and I hope that she made the right decision. I hope her father also believed that God wanted him to live out his days on a machine, that every second of life is sacrosanct. It is certainly possible. And yet I was highly concerned that the daughter was laying the responsibility for her father on God because she couldn't handle it herself.

This experience is a common one in medicine, and we doctors have developed a shortcut for information transfer. In cases where religion is clearly a factor in the decision-making process, one doctor may sign a case out to another using air quotes: They're "waiting for a miracle." In other words, it's not worth talking about goals of care; this family wants everything. And the doctor shuts down, shakes her head, and hoists the patient aboard the end-of-life conveyor belt. I have done this myself many times, even in the case of Mr. Dreux. But of course shortcuts are never a good substitute for careful evaluation of each case.

At a recent meeting of the American Academy of Hospice and Palliative Medicine (AAHPM), I heard a compelling lecture by an African American pastor from the north side of Chicago. He opened his talk with numbers, counting up all of the hours that a God-fearing person in his parish has spent in church over the course of her life. It was a lot. Then he described what is talked about during those hours in church. It's all about hope, he told us. For change, for a better future, for justice, for relief of suffering. And then he asked the predominantly white audience why we expected our African American patients to give up hope— for a cure, for another chance at life—at this most vulnerable point in their lives. This is a time, he said, when they need hope the most.

If the doctor's only concept of hope and miracles is the cure of disease, then there truly is nothing more to talk about with a family wanting everything done in the name of God. But guided by Betty Clark, the pastor on our palliative care team, I have found other ways of transmitting hope to families looking for a miracle. The miracle of time at home, of pain management, of improved quality of life. These are all concepts I have seen families embrace in place of survival—the only concept of hope previously imagined.

I have also found it helpful to open up the question of God's will. Once, a religious family explained to me that they didn't want to play God by withdrawing the breathing tube from their dying loved one. I asked them whether another interpretation might be that they were playing God by keeping her alive when her body was actively dying. Mightn't this be God demonstrating that it was her time to die? And were we, in our hubris, thwarting God's will? Many families agreed with my suggestion that almighty God doesn't need help from mere mortals. If He wants to heal a body, He can do it on his own.

I recognize the complexity of this terrain because I have negotiated it within my own community. I am a practicing Jew. I attend synagogue most Saturdays, and I generally believe there is a greater power in the universe than chance. Given the notion of the sanctity of life in the Torah and the Talmud, the strictest interpretations of Jewish law prohibit the removal of any treatment keeping a patient alive. Clearly, that is not my own belief, nor that of mainstream medical ethics, which supports the withholding and withdrawing of life-support treatments for patients who do not wish to remain dependent on machines.

A few years ago I was asked to lead a Death Cafe alongside my rabbi as a synagogue fund-raiser. Death Cafes have become somewhat of a movement over the past few years. At them, people gather in a nonthreatening environment to consider their own goals of care, learn how to communicate with a health care team, and talk about death and dying. My synagogue is recognized for being particularly diverse; some congregants adhere strictly to Jewish law while others lean more toward the secular. I liked the idea of participating, but I worried that my philosophy of end-of-life care might clash with that of my rabbi. As the leader of this community, he was responsible for presenting congregants with the formal Orthodox Jewish perspective on this topic.

I arranged a meeting with my rabbi and laid out my concerns. "I'm not sure that you will feel comfortable with what I have to say about life support," I said. He listened to my concerns quietly. When I was finished, he said, "I think we're a lot more aligned than you might expect."

We agreed to do the Death Cafe together and to present the various options, including withholding and withdrawing treatments, with the rabbi highlighting approaches most closely aligned with Jewish law, or Halacha. I was surprised at the number and diversity of people who signed up for the Death Cafe: newlyweds, young families, baby boomers, and elderly people. In this public forum, my rabbi and I held different positions. I maintained the position of mainstream bioethics, and my rabbi could agree only partly. But we answered questions and encouraged people to think about how they wanted to run their own lives—and deaths.

It was a stressful moment, to stand before my congregation and say what I believe: that Jewish law has not yet fully accounted for the last century's technological capabilities to keep bodies alive in new, often gruesome ways. And I was well received, by my congregational rabbis as well as by other rabbis in the greater community. *If this age-old religion of mine can adapt to the modern realities of life,* I thought, *then so can the secular world.* I left feeling optimistic.

Weeks after the Death Cafe, my friend Susan, who had attended, called me. "I have a huge favor to ask you," she said. She told me that she worried there would be conflict in her family if her parents ended up dying in an intensive care unit. "I've decided to go to Chicago and sit down with my parents and sister, and I need you to tell me what to say," she said.

Susan was more religiously observant than her parents and

sister, which meant she was uncomfortable with the idea of withdrawing treatments that might keep a parent alive. Yet she felt that her parents' beliefs mattered most here. She realized that her idea of a Jewish death might not be shared by her parents. And what if she and her sister began to argue over a parent's deathbed?

We discussed the possible scenarios and she thought carefully about how she might support her parents' wishes if they were not compatible with her own. When she returned from Chicago, she called me. Her experience had been profoundly positive, she said. The four of them had stayed up late, talking about life, death, and what mattered most to each of them. They laughed and cried. And she left with the sense that she and her sister now had the information they needed to support their parents' wishes.

Food

Almost all of the patients I encounter come from worlds where food is evocative of love and care. Indeed, I can't think of a culture for which this is not true. And in the face of death and suffering, many families see food as a major form of support, both physical and spiritual, for their loved one. Yet this is not the case. Food can be the worst thing to give a dying patient. It burdens an already overloaded system, stopping up the gears, bringing discomfort and suffering to the dying process. When people are actively dying, they almost never want to eat. Yet loving family members will sometimes force food on them—and can feel hurt and desperate if it is not accepted. This may drive an unnecessary wedge between patients and their families at a precious time.

MY PATIENT WAS a seventy-year-old Cantonese-speaking woman with aggressive ovarian cancer. She had been receiving hopeful chemotherapy from her oncologist, but it clearly hadn't been working. On her most recent clinic visit, she was so critically ill that her doctor abruptly admitted her to the ICU for stabilization. He also decided to withhold chemotherapy, to the family's consternation.

Until recently, the cancer had lived quietly inside her, preparing its attack slowly and without raising much alarm. This time, though, it had risen up to fight its final, multifront battle. Fluid around her lungs squeezed like the worst kind of corset, every breath exhausting her. Cancerous fronds curled around her intestines, distending her abdomen and further compromising her breathing.

The first time I met this patient, her son was at her side, feeding her as though she were a little baby. A hospital-cafeteria-issued tuna fish sandwich sat atop a soggy swatch of cellophane on the palm of his left hand. In his right was a butter knife that he used to excise tiny chunks of the sandwich. As I entered the room, he proudly gestured to the remaining portion of the sandwich and communicated reassuringly in broken English that he would keep working hard to get the whole sandwich into his mother. He was part of our team, and his job, he implied, was to contribute to the project of healing his dying mother by nourishing her with love and calories. She lay there, barely able to breathe, intestines obstructed to bursting, every line on her face reading defeat.

Family members frequently feed my patients food, but it is never just food. It is "lumpia, just like he likes it, with roasted pork" or a "mole chicken burrito, not too spicy this time." Beginning with mother's milk, food is not only physical sustenance but spiritual and emotional too. It is a pan-cultural symbol of love, from Chinese and Ethiopian to Jewish and Vietnamese. The dishes have been carefully and lovingly prepared to bring a taste of home into a sterile and frightening place. They are meant as signs of hope, of love and reassurance. Not only for the patient, but for the feeder, too.

And yet for all living things, there comes a time when food becomes something different, something unwelcome, even harmful. An obstructed intestine cannot accommodate a tuna fish sandwich. Even chicken broth, the universal healer of all ills, can increase the pressure in the stomach, causing nausea, vomiting, and stomach pain as well as impeding breathing.

That this elderly Chinese woman was being fed a tuna fish sandwich by her son attested to the desperation he likely felt at that moment. Hospital tuna fish sandwiches are not the food of choice for elderly women from the Chinese mainland. He was caught off guard by her abrupt transfer from the outpatient oncology clinic into the intensive care unit. I imagined he hadn't had time to prepare a special dish.

The patient's face showed sheer exhaustion as her worried son pushed bite after bite into her mouth. Her body had lost the ability to process it, and hunger was a thing of the past. Yet her son was desperate to love her, and this was all he knew how to do.

Worried, I gently coaxed the sandwich away from him. He nodded vigorously as I tried to explain the risk of feeding. But I couldn't climb our Tower of Babel. I made the universal "I'll be right back" sign and ran off to find an interpreter.

As it turned out, he couldn't stop himself from continuing to feed her. Before I had found an interpreter, I heard the familiar words crackling over the PA: "Code Blue, fifth floor." She had indeed aspirated the sandwich. Her already strangled lungs had been filled with what is often a toxin for a dying body—food.

In feeding our dying loved ones, we are feeding ourselves, warding off our own fear of loss. But when physical life begins to pass, we must learn to transfer our love and support into a different medium. The tuna fish sandwich was a desperate act from a desperate son who wanted to love and honor his mother. But his effort may in fact have shortened her life and caused unintended distress and suffering. Whether it's a bowl of grits, matzo ball soup, or a cafeteria tuna fish sandwich, there is a point when food stops being love and starts being dangerous.

Artificial Love

When a person is unable to take food by mouth, life-sustaining calories suspended in liquid are usually infused directly into the stomach through a plastic tube. And feeding tubes function like any of the other plastic tubes we use to prolong life—they keep the body going. Breathing tubes push oxygenated air into a patient's lungs, the dialysis catheters transport the patient's blood to a filter to remove impurities. Sometimes the feeding tube is temporary and travels into the body through the nose or the mouth to descend into the stomach. Other times, it is surgically implanted through the abdominal wall into the stomach, bypassing the throat and neck altogether.

But unlike purely medical interventions, which are already difficult to withdraw once they are shown not to be helping, there is an added layer of difficulty when it comes to feeding tubes. These artificial calories: are they a medical treatment or are they love? And so even with the understanding that this artificial nutrition can actually harm our loved one or make him uncomfortable, families have a hard time letting it go.

This reluctance can even play a role when the family expects the patient to die imminently. In most ventilated patients, the breathing and feeding tubes are entwined together in a patient's mouth before descending into the chest cavity along different paths, one into the lungs, the other into the stomach. Therefore, when the decision has been made to extubate, we usually remove both tubes at once, because of the physical difficulty of separating them and also because we know that continued artificial nutrition would be of no clinical benefit and would indeed cause complications in a patient who is imminently dying.

But it took me several years to realize that it is critical to prepare families in advance for the fact that the feeding tube will no longer be present. Usually this is a moot issue. No longer receiving breathing support, many dying patients cease breathing over minutes, hours, or sometimes days. But occasionally a patient doesn't die as quickly as we predict. Not often, but it happens. Sometimes the patient remains alive three days, five days, even a week after removal of the breathing tube, breathing faintly, blood pressure so low as to be barely palpable. It's at that point that families can start to worry. They begin to notice, unless it has been previously discussed, that there is no feeding tube. Maybe there are no fluids being administered. And they panic. "Shouldn't you be feeding her?"

In the face of this primal anxiety, it is hard for loved ones to hear that administering calories will make things worse. The distrust has been kindled. What kind of doctor wouldn't provide this most basic treatment?

And so now, before withdrawing any tubes, I speak with the family about the lack of benefit of artificial nutrition during the dying process. I tell them that we can never know exactly what day the patient will die. Sometimes we'll be off by a few days, maybe even a week. I have found that this advance preparation helps people to remain calm in the face of withholding nutrition and encourages them to find another way to show their love.

A PATIENT I WORKED WITH several years ago had dementia and could no longer swallow. The intricate workings of the muscles of her throat were failing, and she wasn't able to move food or liquids reliably into her stomach. Instead, they too frequently ended up in her lungs, and she drowned a little with every swallow. She was admitted to my intensive care service with pneumonia from aspirated food that had turned the bottom part of her left lung into a wet sponge. Her blood oxygen levels had dropped so low that we had to support her breathing on a machine.

Now, after being on powerful antibiotics and life support for three days, her oxygen level had improved and her fevers had abated. She was getting better, in a manner of speaking.

This pneumonia was her third, and easily her worst, in four months. This pattern is typical of end-stage dementia, when patients commonly lose control of their swallowing mechanism and often die from pneumonias resulting from food lodging in the lung. Usually, these patients have gone in and out of the hospital through a sort of revolving door; as soon as one pneumonia is chased away by antibiotics, another emerges.

The option of a feeding tube had been offered to this patient's family when she was admitted to the emergency room. "If she makes it through this, she should get a feeding tube so that it doesn't happen again," they were told. And so now that she was improving, her family was asking for the tube.

But contrary to popular belief, a feeding tube does not prolong life in a patient with advanced dementia. It actually increases suffering. A stomach full of mechanically pumped artificial calories puts pressure on an already fragile digestive system, increasing the chance of pushing stomach contents up into the lungs. And surgically implanted tubes are a setup for complications: dislodgement, bleeding, and infections that can result in pain, hospital admissions, and the use of arm restraints on already confused patients. But maybe most important, the medical-

EXTREME MEASURES

ization of food deprives the dying of some of the last remnants of the human experience: taste, smell, touch, and connection to loved ones.

So why do so many demented patients die with feeding tubes?

As I've already stated, food is how we know best to care for one another, from breast to deathbed. And thus to stop feeding runs contrary to every impulse we have as humans. Even for doctors. As a dying person becomes unable to process food on her own, our tendency is to plug life into her with a tube pumping artificial nutrition.

Yet for millennia we humans have fed our dying by hand. Spooned slowly so as not to overwhelm, a trickle of broth or a favorite food ground up to taste were the last small pleasures for a dying body. We fed until they would take no more and knew that we had done everything we could. But with the feeding tube, we can keep going. Patients frequently die with plastic tubes weaving mysteriously under their gowns, entering their bodies at unnatural angles, rendering them a little more alien to us. Those who are most needed sit a little farther away from the bed, afraid to dislodge tubes that are supposedly keeping their loved one alive. And the patient's mouth will usually remain dry and empty until the end.

My last conversation about the patient's feeding took place on my way to my car Friday afternoon. The patient's sister was walking in as I was walking out. She thanked me for the care I'd provided and told me that, despite my recommendations, the family had decided to go with the tube. "I couldn't not feed her," she said. "I can't leave her starving."

The next day, my patient was wheeled down to the operating room for her feeding tube, then a few hours later wheeled back to intensive care. Over the next couple of weeks, her sister sat with her most days, wearing the requisite paper gown and gloves for guests of patients with resistant bacteria from prolonged hospital stays. She sat off to the side, separated from her sister by tubes, bedrails, and the bustle of activity around them. The patient died two weeks later in the intensive care unit, a different pneumonia in her lungs.

In the face of death, food can feel like life—and hope. But it is our job to remember that in most cases it is neither.

A Sense of Duty

Another powerful factor when it comes to medical decision making at the end of life is the weight of social obligation. A dying person may feel obligated to conform to another's goals in order to fulfill a social role or a sense of duty. Whether in the role of parent, child, spouse, or elder, I have seen patients defer their own needs in order to offer solace to someone close to them.

Mr. Saephan was a seventy-nine-year-old man with dying kidneys. He'd been urinating less and less frequently, and over the past several weeks his breathing had become increasingly labored. He was brought into the ER by his worried family late Friday night. There, labs showed that his blood was filled with acid from kidney failure, and his lungs were full of fluid that could not be released as urine. He was agitated, delirious, and very short of breath. The ER staff intubated him for low oxygen levels and sent him to the ICU.

The ICU team inserted a temporary catheter and emergency dialysis was started. Over the next several days, following the removal of several liters of fluid and dialysis, he improved. His breathing tube was removed and he was able to breathe easily on his own. His delirium and anxiety lifted.

Early in the patient's hospitalization, the family had consented to surgical placement of a fistula—the tying together of large blood vessels to provide a stable port of entry for the dialysis catheter, a common technique used in chronic dialysis. But the patient, now awake and off the ventilator, surprised the team by refusing the procedure. He didn't want it, he told them.

His family was upset, but he was firm. I was called in as the palliative care consultant by the team to discuss his goals of care and to help the family process this change of course. At his side was his grandson Tommy, a twenty-year-old student at a local junior college. He wore a hospital-issued yellow gown to protect against his grandfather's resistant bacterial colonies and a blue bouffant cap sitting low on his forehead, as if he didn't have the energy to push it up. He sat without talking or moving, save for handing his grandfather the telephone when it rang, which was often, each time with a different relative eager to send good wishes. At the end of the call, Tommy would hang up the phone quietly and sit waiting for the next.

I introduced myself with the Mien interpreter. The patient nodded politely. Tommy sat tentative and quiet but unmoving. I explained my purpose, that I was here to talk to the patient about his understanding of the situation and to help him think through next steps. I asked Mr. Saephan if he would prefer to speak about these issues in private to start with. Tommy sat motionless beside him. The patient appeared to be considering it.

Seconds passed, more than was comfortable, and I asked again whether the patient would prefer to speak alone. After a sidelong glance at his unmoving grandson, the patient shrugged permission for Tommy to remain in the room.

I asked Mr. Saephan about himself. About what he understood of his illness. He knew that his kidneys were failing and had almost caused his death. He understood that we had started dialysis on an emergency basis, rescuing him from the brink of death. "I know that dialysis won't fix my kidneys," he said to me, his tone a combination of a question and answer. I explained that it was true, it would not fix them, merely take over the role of cleaning his blood. He nodded quietly. That was what he feared, he said.

He began to tell me about his friends who had been on dialysis. He had watched them become shriveled and weak, he said, with constant nausea. He had watched them become dependent on family members to take them to the dialysis center three times a week where they were attached to metal boxes, which whirred and sucked at them for several hours. He suspected the machines had sucked their power away. In his large family, he had always been the "strong one," the patriarch, the decision maker. While he wanted to be there for them, he didn't want to live this way.

He became more animated as he talked and actually sat up in bed a little more, leaning toward me, his skinny arms on his bony knees. I then asked him what he would choose for himself if he had no one to answer to, no one depending on him. Without hesitation, he leaned closer to me and said, "I would stop this." He held up the end of his Quinton catheter in explanation.

At that moment, I heard a sniffle. Tommy had been silent this whole time, quiet as a mouse. I'd actually forgotten about him, and so, apparently, had Mr. Saephan. As we both turned toward him, a large tear, just one, welled up and spilled down his cheek.

Tommy made no move to wipe it away. Without missing a beat, Mr. Saephan turned his face back to me and said, "But I need to keep living. For my family."

He lay back in the bed and closed his eyes.

EXTREME MEASURES

There are innumerable ways that our backgrounds can influence our preferences and behavior—far too many ever to include here. But all of them, from the most self-evident to the subtlest, remind me that the human being is unknowable—unless maybe you ask.

chapter six

Who We Are

THE PATIENT WAS AN eighty-five-year-old man who had been diagnosed with lung cancer one year ago. When I met him, it had already metastasized to his brain and bones. He did not believe in Western medicine and had refused the biopsy that the oncologist recommended as well as any treatment for the cancer. He was admitted to our ICU with a complete left lung collapse caused by an enlarging lesion. His kidneys were failing fast. His blood pressure was flagging. The man would have died were it not for the machines and medicines keeping him going.

I was on the palliative care service when we received the call to come and help with the case. The resident calling in the consult was a bit vague. I couldn't tell what the actual consultation question was. When I began to read the chart, I realized that what they really needed most was our support for their own moral distress. They were concerned that they were treating the patient against his will.

There was profound family dysfunction, I was told, and the team felt that the patient's older son had anointed himself decision maker against the wishes of the patient's daughter, who had been caring for the patient until this point. This apparent coup was all the more concerning because the son was suspected by the team to have a serious personality disorder. It was rumored that the daughter had taken out a restraining order against her brother. And the son was now ordering the team to keep his father alive at all costs, a treatment plan that seemed at odds with everything we were finding out about the patient.

Dr. Danforth, a member of the ethics committee, filled me in further. There was ample evidence from the oncologist, the patient's daughter, and other family members that the patient was not inclined toward intensive treatments, or even Western medicine. He had begged to go home from the hospital on several occasions during various admissions, and he had clearly told Dr. Raj, the oncologist who had made the original diagnosis, that he didn't want to be kept alive on machines without a chance of recovery. Dr. Raj had in fact signed a Physician Order for Life-Sustaining Treatment (POLST), ordering that the patient not be placed on a breathing machine or receive CPR. But, Dr. Raj told the ethics committee, the son had convinced the patient to rescind the order. And now all of this patient's worst fears were being realized as he hurtled toward death while strapped to a bed in our ICU.

I told Dr. Danforth that I would meet with the son that afternoon and try to understand what was going on. Dr. Danforth said he would come to provide support. This situation seemed as if it had the potential to explode.

The meeting was scheduled for 2 P.M., but the son arrived an hour late, as was his habit. By then, our Cantonese interpreter was waiting, along with the patient's daughter. She and her estranged brother stood shifting uncomfortably as I opened the door to the conference room. We entered the cold room, and everyone took a seat—the daughter in a distant corner, the son at the center of the table, stretched out as if he owned the place. Dr. Danforth sat in a corner, observing.

Something about the son struck me as off. He was overly animated for such a somber moment, even jaunty. He shook hands with every person in our group and made small talk through the interpreter. I had the sense of watching an entertainer, or even a politician, and struggled to connect with the human behind the façade. His sister, meanwhile, sat quietly in the corner of the room, hunched over the purse on her lap.

I asked him what he understood about his father's condition. He told us through the interpreter that he knew his father was very sick. But he was a fighter, he said. His father wanted to live.

"You're right that he's very sick," I said. "Our oncologists and radiation doctors say that there is no further treatment that can make him better. He is days from death." From what I knew about his father, I said, he didn't strike me as the type of man who would want to die with a plastic tube in his mouth. I listed all of the evidence I had before me to support that conjecture. I then went on to recommend that we switch goals of care now, remove the breathing tube, and attend to any suffering before he died.

The room was silent. The son blinked behind his fashionable glasses. I found myself wondering why we had allowed this man to drive his father's care. But there it was. The squeaky wheel gets the grease.

The son turned to the interpreter and began to explain again, with great confidence, that his father had wanted to stay alive at all costs. The daughter sat forward in her chair. She looked ready to pounce on him.

"Father didn't want this," she said steadily, her lips tight. "He told me that he didn't want to be on machines if he couldn't get better."

They started to bicker. Our interpreter looked up at me and shrugged. "I cannot really keep up. But he keeps telling her that he is recording the conversation to use in court."

The son was large. And intimidating. He stood up and moved toward his tiny sister, punctuating his words in loud staccato. Watching this scene and remembering the rumored restraining order made me fear for the daughter's safety. It was time to stop the conversation. Emotions were flaring, and I had a strong feeling that the yelling match was not about the question at hand but about something much more primal, and certainly unsolvable by a doctor and her interpreter sitting in a conference room as the father lay dying.

I didn't have an answer for the team. And the ethics committee didn't have an answer for me. If, as everyone seemed to agree, there was ample evidence that this patient's will was being violated, then we were obligated to change the current goals of care from life prolongation to extubation and comfort management. But it is very difficult to stand up against an intimidating person who claims to have legal surrogate status. Especially when he seems a bit off balance and is invoking lawyers and restraining orders.

In the end, I was able to do the right thing. Backed by the primary team and the ethics committee, I sucked in a breath, put on my poker face, and calmly told the son that we would be disconnecting his father from the breathing machine. I understood his disappointment, I said, but we doctors had decided that the evidence was clear. This would not be what his father would have wanted.

This case ended as well as it could. He nodded and walked out of the ICU, never to return. But it might have been different. He might have been violent, litigious, or just plain mean. And those possibilities can be extremely daunting to a physician trying her best to do the right thing.

If my formal medical education only minimally addressed culture and religion, there was almost nothing when it came to the psychological and social factors at play within families at the end of life. Personality disorders, anxiety and depression, cognitive limitations, financial motivations—these are but some of the issues that can derail a patient-centered process. I have come to recognize certain patterns over the years, even as I am consistently reminded that every person and family system is unique.

Family Dysfunction

In *Anna Karenina*, Leo Tolstoy famously wrote: "All happy families are alike; each unhappy family is unhappy in its own way." There is no time like the death of a loved one for family dysfunction to play itself out. A dying parent can trigger old traumas, revive old guilts and betrayals. Birth order, inheritance, sibling rivalry: These are but a few of the issues that have impacted decision making in my patients' lives.

There are as many roadblocks to good decision making as there are patients and families. One common prototype is "the sister who flew in from the coast"—doctor code for a family member who arrives at the eleventh hour on a mission to rally forces to save her loved one, often disrupting a carefully considered care plan. This is often someone who hasn't seen her parent regularly or participated in the past weeks of decision making.

When she gets to the bedside, she cannot abide the decision to allow a natural death. She insists that everything be done, and levels criticisms at the family members and doctors who have been at ground zero. Maybe it's her own guilt. Maybe it's sibling rivalry. Maybe it's simply grief at the loss of a parent, or a combination of all of these. But once the conflict is in the room, it's virtually impossible to smooth it over. The stakes ratchet up quickly and people polarize.

There are many other reasons why the de facto decision maker isn't the right person to make decisions for a seriously ill loved one. Even if that person truly is next of kin, she may not be interested, able, or appropriate in that role. A spouse who has been separated from the patient for years. A daughter who suffered sexual abuse by the patient. A son who will continue to benefit from his father's Social Security checks. A parent whose guilt or grief impedes clear decision making. But sometimes there is no one else to work with and we have no choice.

Even if there are no such issues, a family member may simply feel uncomfortable in the role of surrogate decision maker. He may feel incapable of or unwilling to speculate on what the patient would choose for herself; no, he might tell me, we never talked about dying or the Terri Schiavo case, never had a sick family member on life support. And then there are those who are clear that their loved one would not want her life artificially prolonged, but feel they cannot make that final decision without explicit instructions from the patient. If there is no family member willing to step up and make a decision, we are in a holding pattern that usually defaults to the end-of-life conveyor belt.

FRED CARTER WAS A ninety-year-old patient with prostate cancer that had metastasized to the vertebrae in his neck. The cancer had ravaged these crucial bones protecting the spinal cord until they were as soft as overcooked chicken bones. He also had mild dementia and was suffering from septic shock from infected urine that could not bypass his swollen prostate.

I met him in our ICU the morning after he had suffered two consecutive cardiac arrests, one at his nursing home and another on admission to our emergency room. During each, he was aggressively resuscitated with chest compressions, electrical shocks, and strong drips to boost his almost nonexistent blood pressure.

He remained critically ill and in a coma, requiring maximal support from the breathing machine and blood pressure medications. After several days, to our astonishment, he woke up—he even stuck out his tongue and blinked on command. But then his neurologic catastrophe revealed itself. When we asked him to squeeze a hand or wiggle his toes, he couldn't. Our well-intentioned resuscitative efforts had crushed his cancer-weakened neck bones, rendering him quadriplegic. He couldn't move any part of his body below the neck. Although he tried to breathe on his own, he couldn't without the machine. His unstable neck made it too dangerous to send him to radiology for an MRI, and even if we could, a surgical fix was almost inconceivable.

It was no one's fault—any doctor or paramedic faced with a patient having a cardiac arrest would be expected to perform this procedure on the patient unless there was documentation that the patient did not want it. There was none.

The patient was now tethered to our machines, completely paralyzed, and awake—a reality that chilled me to the bone. He would never again breathe on his own, and we needed to decide about traching him for permanent ventilator support. Our social worker had not yet found any family, which happens regularly in our ICU. But according to a note from his previous hospitalization weeks before, he had been alert enough to make his own treatment decisions despite his mild dementia. I decided to give it a try.

I asked him to wiggle his toes; I wasn't sure if he realized yet that he no longer had the ability to do so.

"Do you notice that you can't move your body?" I asked. He gave a slight nod.

I took a deep breath.

"I am concerned that this is permanent," I said. Those were hard words to say. Harder, of course, to hear.

No response.

I waited. He was trapped. Even if he wanted to ask a question, it would be extremely difficult. He could move nothing except his facial muscles and seemed somewhat disoriented. I decided to keep the information flowing in the hopes that it might elicit some sign of preference regarding placement of a trach. I said, "You're ninety years old." And then, although it felt awful, I asked him if he'd thought about his own death.

He stared at me but again gave no response. I rephrased, re-framed. Still, nothing.

Up to this point in the hospitalization, and despite multiple calls by our social worker, there hadn't been any family to talk to. But later that day, a son showed up. He was the first of many to come over the following days. The patient, originally from South Carolina, had had children with a few different women— it was unclear exactly how many. Most now lived in California. Several were meeting each other for the first time at the bedside. A widening circle accumulated as the news grew that their father was in the hospital. These meetings didn't have the feel of a fam-ily reunion, but rather a contest over who was closest, most ap-propriate to make decisions, most entitled to inherit his house.

There was a woman thirty years his junior who I was told was his wife. Later, it turned out she was "just a girlfriend." She had been living elsewhere for several years and returned to the area when she heard he was hospitalized. "She isn't really involved," I was told by one of the sons. And yet at the first big family meeting they all called her Mama, which confused me. She was in possession of an Advance Directive from his last hospitalization stating that she was the surrogate decision maker for any major medical decisions. But it wasn't notarized properly, as was pointed out to me by the social worker and the patient's eldest son. I was told about a piece of property that two of the sons had started fighting over months earlier.

I was being pulled into private family meetings left and right by various parties. I didn't know with whom I should talk. The patient, while appearing alert, was not attempting to communicate at all. Who should be the decision maker? Who was the right surrogate, legally and ethically? I was worried that the people I was talking to weren't necessarily concerned with the patient's best interest. Two of his sons from different marriages said they believed he wouldn't want to be kept alive like this. Others said he was a fighter. But, finally, those involved agreed he would not want to be surgically attached to a machine. We set a date to extubate him, but that date got pushed back, and then pushed back again as I tried to accommodate for as much consensus as possible.

I arranged for another meeting, another attempt to corral this growing mass of people into formulating a clear plan for this man. Twenty-three people showed up. Two babies, one at the breast. I went through the grim medical realities, explaining his critical condition as well as the fact that he was trapped—awake but unlikely ever to move again.

"But he's so alert," said one relative, "what will it look like when the tube comes out and he can't continue to breathe on his own?"

I acknowledged that these types of cases were the hardest for me, when the patient was awake and responsive to his family. Disconnecting the breathing machine, which would likely result in immediate death, felt like too much responsibility. But, I said, the alternative is to keep him attached to the machines until he dies, which could be days, weeks, even months. And, for some patients, that might be a fate worse than death.

They decided against removing him from the machines without his input. I described my previous attempts but agreed that it made sense to try again. I recommended that we keep the group small and quiet, and that I use a simple and carefully scripted set of questions in order to enable clear communication. They refused, insisting that every one of them gown and glove up and be present for the conversation. And they wanted to ask the questions. "Because he's more likely to respond to Denise than to you," I was told. Denise was one of his daughters. The Reverend Miller, a hospital chaplain, was at the meeting and offered support for my approach, but they would have none of it. They marched toward the room en masse. I followed behind, the reverend's hand supportive on my arm.

The medical student's note gives a detailed description of one of the most dysfunctional decision-making processes I have ever seen. The family gathered around the bedside of this critically ill, newly quadriplegic ninety-year-old man. Denise asked the patient five times if he wanted the tube out of his mouth. He nodded each time. The room was filled with excited murmuring, but Denise wasn't convinced. She switched her approach. "You'll die if we take this out. Do you want to die?" This time he did not respond. "See, he wants to keep it in," she said. There was some clapping.

I leaned toward the reverend. "I guess if I try to ask him again, they'll accuse me of murder," I whispered.

"Yes," he said, "don't even try."

I went off service that day and signed the case out to the subsequent attending physician. The following week, I heard, the patient suffered a massive stroke and was no longer responsive. The family decided at that point to remove the breathing tube and the patient died shortly thereafter.

With a decision-making committee this large, complex, and filled with conflict, a vulnerable patient is at risk of being shunted out of the center of the process. And there are times when we doctors, despite our best intentions, can only stand by and watch.

Diminished Capacity

Enrique spent every day by his wife's side, holding her bruised and swollen hands, listening to the swish of the breathing machine. They had been married for more than thirty years, a close, comfortable relationship. Now he sat quietly next to her, day after day, his uneaten lunch in a neat bag beside his feet, waiting for her to wake up.

But she never would.

Clara, a janitor at a local hospital, had been at home mopping the kitchen floor when her heart stopped. By the time the paramedics arrived, she had been without oxygen for twelve minutes, a lifetime for tender brain tissue. Now she was in the ICU, her lungs inflating and deflating to the rhythm of the mechanical ventilator, blood oxygen level reading normal. But she was completely unresponsive. Her brain had been starved of oxygen for too long. "Prognosis is extremely poor for significant clinical improvement," read the neurologists' sixth and final note. "We will sign off for now. Please don't hesitate to call us back if anything changes." Clara would probably never eat, smile, or move voluntarily again. But it takes time for us to be sure—and thus the family still had room to hope.

Enrique was the picture of the devoted husband. When the doctors first came in the room and saw him next to Clara's bed holding her hand, his eyes red from crying, they addressed him as the surrogate decision maker. He was, after all, the patient's husband. Clara's three sisters were often in the room as well. They each bore a striking similarity to the intubated patient, and I was told that the four women had been extremely close. They had talked to each other several times per day by phone.

For most of that first week, the sisters stood quietly in the back of the room as the team spoke to Enrique, listening carefully to all that he said—or didn't. Each time the team met with him to explain Clara's poor prognosis, he would nod, smile, and thank the team.

"She will be all right," he would say, smiling. "God will make it so."

By the beginning of the second week, as the doctors were becoming clearer on the poor prognosis, the sisters were less likely to stand quietly and listen to Enrique. They had begun to disagree, sometimes vehemently, with him. The palliative care team was invited into the case to assist with the brewing conflict and help identify goals of care. Like the medical team, they noticed that Enrique didn't seem to be processing, or perhaps even comprehending, the information given him. After performing some informal capacity assessments, they became concerned that he might not be the appropriate decision maker; he didn't seem to understand basic concepts about Clara's prognosis, the impact of treatment options, or the process of substituted decision making. When the team asked him about Clara's personality, values, or preferences, he repeatedly responded with his own, despite our repeated reminders that it was Clara we needed to focus upon.

Most states have a rank order of surrogate legitimacy. A spouse is considered the most legitimate, then adult children, then other relatives. California is unusual in that it is one of the few states allowing the person most familiar with the patient's values to act as surrogate, regardless of traditional rank order.

In the beginning, Clara's sisters had taken care of Enrique— bringing food to him in the hospital, doing his laundry, cleaning the house. It was what Clara would have wanted, they said. When the sisters began to understand that Clara would never wake up again, this began to shift.

That is when they told us they knew without a doubt Clara would not want to be kept alive in this condition. She had told them herself, in detail, instructing each of them repeatedly to ensure that she was never kept alive on machines. She was unusually savvy about these preferences, given her work in the hospital as well as her own medical history. Clara had been living with a heart condition for years and had envisioned this very cardiac arrest. She had seen cardiac arrest patients with poor neurologic function in the ICU on machines, she told her sisters, and she would never want to live like that herself. And now, the sisters told us, her husband was overriding her wishes.

Enrique had worked for years on an assembly line in a sponge factory. The couple had no children. Clara took care of Enrique as if he were her son. He didn't even know how to use an ATM, the sisters told the doctors. Enrique's only duty was to go back and forth to his shift at the sponge factory and bring home a small paycheck. Without her he was lost, they said.

By now the sisters were avoiding Enrique and coming to the hospital less frequently. It wasn't because they didn't want to see their dear sister, brush her hair, stroke her arm, they told us. Rather, it was because they had grown to hate their brother-in-law. They would visit only when they knew he would not be there.

In the end, Clara was plugged into machines. The palliative care team had been actively trying to switch decision-making capacity over to the sisters, but this is a slow process, and in the meantime, a new team had come on service. They found Clara beginning her third week with a temporary breathing tube, now overdue for removal. The surgeons had an unexpected opening on the operating room list. Enrique was in the room. He signed the papers for the trach.

Personal Value System

Bobby Hancock was sixty-two years young and very involved in his community. He worked at the local flea market by day and was a jazz musician by night. Over the previous two months, he told us, he had lost thirty pounds without trying. He had come to the emergency room a few days earlier with nausea, vomiting, and abdominal pain. The CT scan showed a large mass obstructing his colon. Food and liquid were unable to pass and had smashed up against the obstruction, causing dilation of the bowel. The CT scan also showed a mass in his liver, worrisome for metastatic disease from the colon, especially given the profound weight loss. If proven by biopsy, this would be a terrible diagnosis. But colon cancer is sometimes responsive to chemotherapy. Maybe, if he was lucky and had the right type, he could live a few more years. But he didn't want what we had to offer. The biopsies, the chemotherapy, maybe even a surgery. The team was growing desperate.

I was called in as the palliative care attending to manage his symptoms and try to get through to him.

His bowel obstruction had largely resolved by the time I met him. He had received a cocktail of medications to shrink the swelling around the tumor and so the trapped fluid had begun to trickle slowly past the obstruction. A tube snaked from his nose into his stomach, sucking some of the obstructing contents northward into a container attached to the wall. With relief of the pressure in his intestines, his profound nausea, vomiting, and abdominal distension had diminished.

The patient smiled politely when I walked into the room and gestured for me to sit. His bed sat next to a dusty window, looking out on scaffolding. A colorful macramé bracelet was loose around his skinny wrist, highlighting how out of place he was in this cold, gray room. I introduced myself to him in the innocuous way that we learn to do in palliative care, identifying myself as an expert in symptom management. Talking about nausea and vomiting is often easier than discussing the implications of life-limiting illness, at least to start. "Thank you very much for fixing my nausea and vomiting," he said, "but I really want to get out of the hospital as soon as I can. No offense, but I don't trust Western medicine."

He told me that he prided himself on living as healthy a life as he could. He neither smoked nor drank, only "a little reefer here and there." He exercised and kept to a vegan diet. He had watched a number of his friends suffer through chronic diseases and cancers, wasting away on machines or chemotherapy, and he harbored a deep distrust of the medical system. He stayed away from doctors at all costs and wasn't going to start seeing them now, he said with some pride.

I was convinced that he didn't really understand the issues. Chemotherapy, I explained, might give him more time, especially

EXTREME MEASURES

given his good functional status. And depending on the exact cell structure that we would see on biopsy, some of the less toxic treatments might work. "I'll never get enough extra time to make it worthwhile," he said. "How about six extra months?" I asked. He shook his head. "A year?" Another shake. "How about two?" He told me he would discuss it with his mother, but that it probably wouldn't make a difference.

Now I realized that it made no sense to keep pushing for a biopsy. Although it might answer our own questions, this man was flat-out refusing all treatments, even those with fewer side effects. "My friends were begging their doctors to keep them alive," he said. "They took all kinds of poisons but they got sicker and sicker. They couldn't even get out of bed. When my time comes, I'm ready," he said.

Okay, I thought. You can't force chemotherapy on someone who doesn't want it. But I worried that he would develop another bowel obstruction soon. And that is a terrible way to die. Nausea, vomiting, abdominal pain. Yet we have ways of avoiding these symptoms—a venting gastrostomy tube allows for removal of air and liquid directly from the stomach through the abdominal wall. In my view, a minor inconvenience compared to a bowel obstruction.

But again he would have none of it. He claimed that he could keep himself from becoming obstructed again by not eating. I explained that that was highly unlikely, since even saliva can build up and contribute to obstruction. But he was firm. "It's disgusting," he said. "Those bags are only for people who are trying to beat the inevitable."

This man was clear. Clear thinking, clear values, clear goals. They may have been different from mine, but he was unshakable. "Once it's in the liver, it's all over," he said. I explained that patients could live with colon cancer, even if it had spread to the liver, sometimes for years. But he just shook his head.

I realized then that my agenda was just that: my agenda. What made sense to me did not work for him. I had done my job by providing him with the clinical information that he deserved. Several times. And he had politely accepted that information and decided against my recommendation. At a certain point, I needed to remember that my values were mine. Not his.

A 2015 study in *JAMA Surgery* revealed that Bobby's instinct had led him in the right direction after all. In this study, younger patients with colon cancer that had metastasized to other organs received significantly more chemotherapy than did older counterparts. Yet they experienced only a minimal gain in survival and a lot more suffering from the toxic chemotherapy. In other words, less may indeed be more. Perhaps Bobby wasn't as far out as we all thought.

The Women of Buttonwood Court

I was invited to give a talk at Buttonwood Court, a local independent living facility. Its end-of-life committee consisted mostly of women in their eighties who had watched their husbands die over the previous several years. They were activists, these aged women, determined to design their own deaths. Some were motivated by having seen bad deaths, others by seeing good ones. What unified them was a drive to be prepared, open, and clearly understood by those who loved them.

I was surprised to learn that almost every one of them had completed a POLST. In fact, they acknowledged it as a badge of honor. This bright pink form documents a patient's specific choices regarding the use of medical technologies such as CPR, breathing machines, and feeding tubes. Unlike an Advance Directive, the POLST is a signed doctor's order. And for those who do not wish to experience cardiopulmonary resuscitation, it is the only legal protection against receiving these otherwise default treatments. First responders like EMTs and paramedics are legally required to use every technique to keep a patient alive unless there is a signed doctor's order to the contrary, even in the presence of protesting family members.

A POLST should not be confused with a DNR order, also signed by a physician, but active only for that particular admission in that particular hospital. A POLST ideally follows the patient wherever he goes, whether to hospitals, nursing homes, or home. It is even transportable across most state lines.

Unfortunately, a paper document like the POLST is flimsy protection against treatments that are so readily performed by well-meaning medical personnel. Given how easily it can be misplaced, lost, or destroyed, some people wear a metal MedicAlert bracelet—recognized in most states as a legal substitute for a POLST—with the appropriate instructions on them.

Although the POLST form has seen recent gains in use, most laypeople have still never heard of it. And at the time that I spoke at Buttonwood Court, even most physicians and social workers were unfamiliar with it. But to me, this form is a powerful tool, the only thing that can shield a person from the life-saving St. Bernards that we health care providers have become.

To my surprise, almost everyone in this audience knew what a POLST form was. In fact, many had already obtained one from a physician, they told me with pride—all with instructions to allow the person to die a natural death if he was found in cardiac or pulmonary arrest. I looked around the room. To be sure, there were walkers parked throughout the audience, a lot of white hair, and some crooked postures . . . but the people who had shown up at this lecture were very much alive. They asked excellent questions, often with humor. They certainly seemed to be enjoying themselves. And their lives.

I started to wonder if they understood what it was they were so adamantly opposed to. Did they realize that the ICU might indeed rescue them from pneumonia or from a lung punctured in a car accident, and very likely put them right back into their lives at Buttonwood Court? Was this unanimity groupthink, the work of a few zealous people who were so opposed to the idea of mechanized deaths that they had not only rejected the ICU in its entirety, but convinced the rest of them too?

I felt that I needed to say something. I wanted them to understand that there was indeed a role for our lifesaving technologies, to tell them of the patients I had cared for who were just like them, old yet vibrant, saved by our treatments and able to go back to living their lives.

But they simply didn't agree. They didn't want to be in my ICU, not one of them. Yes, they said, we are happy to be alive right now. We have friends, an active life of the mind, children, and grandchildren to see on weekends and holidays. Most of us are relatively healthy for our age, with no great suffering or pain. The food at Buttonwood Court is delicious and our apartments have lovely views. The problem with the ICU, they said, is that it takes away control; it increases the risk of being hijacked into the prolonged death that every one of us has pledged to avoid.

In the end, we agreed to disagree. As it stands now for me, if I were a healthy elder, I would be willing to give the ICU a time-limited trial to see if it could turn my pneumonia or serious urinary tract infection around. But the women of Buttonwood Court did teach me something important. Sometimes it isn't that the doctor needs to work harder to elicit the patient's values but that those values are simply different from the doctor's. Yet another lesson in listening.

. . .

THEN THERE WAS VERONICA SANTOS, who also eschewed the principles of Western medicine. She'd been diagnosed eight years earlier with localized, hormone-responsive breast cancer. As cancer goes, this is considered a desirable diagnosis, often curable with surgery and relatively mild chemotherapy. But unchecked, it spreads like any other cancer.

Veronica was a physical therapist. She prided herself on her understanding of the health care system and all that it lacked: its false promises, the suffering within its walls, the toxic chemicals. At the time of her diagnosis, she had decided to pursue only naturopathic treatments, she told me. Acupuncture, herbs, and meditation, for starters. There were two trips to Mexico to visit *curanderas*, or traditional healers. For eight years, she had avoided any contact with Western medicine. Until now. A violent sneeze had shattered her cancer-ridden pelvis. There were no real surgical options. She was unable to move and was in excruciating pain in the bed. It hurt, she told me, to smile.

I fully anticipated that she would reject any offer of treatments aimed at her cancer. But when she balked at my recommendation for medications and treatments that could treat her pain and stabilize the bone destruction, decreasing the possibility of more fractures, I was at a loss. The data were unequivocal. These interventions—bisphosphonate medication and radiation therapy—provided benefits with minimal burdens, even for those patients approaching the end of life. Bisphosphonates had less than a 1 percent risk of complications and could be provided by hospice services in her home every month. Radiation therapy, which we could perform in one session before she left hospital, conveyed a similarly favorable benefit-to-burden ratio for patients like Veronica. Although these treatments wouldn't cure the cancer, they would stabilize her bones and provide some relief. She agreed to look over some reading about both therapies and asked me to come back and talk to her later. In the meantime, she reluctantly agreed to take some pain medications but asked that we keep it at the lowest possible dose. She was bedridden with a shattered pelvis, and I shuddered to imagine how she must be feeling with each bed turn or attempt to void urine or stool.

In the end, she agreed to the bisphosphonates but not to the radiation therapy. She wanted to go home right away with hospice and looked forward to continuing her herbal supplements and (she whispered) medical marijuana. If the pain got really bad, she assured me, she would use the ibuprofen. I practically begged her to take home a bottle of oral morphine. She conceded, but I don't think she had any intention of using it.

My time with Veronica was eye opening. As I've discussed, most patients at the end of life want too much care, and for that, they suffer. But I worry that Veronica held a contrary but equally chilling belief: that the traditional health care system had nothing to offer her in her final days.

As the old adage says, everything in moderation. It seems to me to be an issue of using what works and avoiding what doesn't. In my opinion, palliative care would have helped Veronica in her final days or weeks. But I can't know for sure. Maybe, for example, sedation from pain medications would have caused her more suffering than the pain itself. I have trouble wrapping my head around that, but she was the one in the bed, not I.

Avoidance and Denial

A good friend of mine is a trust and estates lawyer. I am struck by the similarities between our work: We both aim to prepare those we serve for the ultimate reality of life—death and dying. And we both encounter resistance.

She tells of clients, more than one would expect, who pay her to draw up documents to protect their estates in the case of their deaths yet never complete the necessary tasks to do so. Sometimes it is just the final signature that is missing, despite her repeated contacts and reminders. She doesn't hear from many of these clients again, even though her bill is almost always paid. Those who do finally respond are sheepish about their procrastination. Some admit that they couldn't bring themselves to sign it. "It just felt too final," is a common refrain. She has conducted at least a dozen deathbed signings, where she is summoned to help a client who may be days, even hours away from death, sign papers she had drafted months before. These patients are fatigued, in pain, and often questionably alert. There are the usual excuses for the delay—doctor's appointments, not feeling up to it—but she suspects that the main cause is simply fear and grief about their own mortality.

She began working with one of her clients when he was eighty-one. A successful businessman, he had built his manufacturing company from the ground up as a young man and was now the CEO and CFO and held all other positions of importance. He had a child from a brief early marriage as well as children from a second marriage and wanted to ensure that his estate would go in very specific proportions to each child. My friend arranged his will accordingly and then went on to do what any good trust and estates attorney would do—help him prepare for the day when he would hand his business and estate over to his children. And so, at their first meeting several years earlier, she said frankly: "What is going to happen to your business and estate when you die?" He appeared flabbergasted, possibly insulted. "I'm healthy. I have many years left." And that was as far as he would go. Not that my friend didn't try. She is used to her clients avoiding these conversations, at least at first. She's learned to push through it, as I have with my patients. These are difficult topics and require fortitude and persistence. "That's why you're paying me," she said. But he would have none of it. Not at that meeting or at the others over the course of years.

At each meeting, she would ask what would happen if he were not available to manage the business. Who knew the passwords, the accounts, even the customers? Wouldn't it make sense to sell the business to the young partner who worked alongside him? "The business is my baby. Would you be willing to give up your baby?"

But then it happened. Everything she had warned him about. A massive stroke. Complete physical dependence requiring a full-time attendant to feed him and keep him clean. And his mind was gone. He could no longer communicate or answer even simple questions. He did not acknowledge the presence of others, if he was aware of them at all. His business went immediately into a downward spiral, losing hundreds of thousands of dollars per month. His children's inheritance shrank with every passing day. And the financial losses were minor compared to what happened to the family itself. The children spent hundreds of hours trying to right the ship. Their frustration with their father was surpassed only by their resentment of one another. The business became embroiled in a lawsuit. A father's denial ended up shattering the family he had intended to protect.

My Own Procrastination

I flew to Florida a while back. Before leaving, I did what I always do before a trip. I gathered up all of the stray junk on my desk in the hope that I might actually get something done on the five-hour flight. Stray medical journals, some bills, camp forms for my kids . . . they all made the cut. And of course the yellow Advance

Directive booklet that had been sitting on my desk for four years, shamefully incomplete. At this point I'm not sure how many trips it has taken with me. I believe it went to Israel last winter break and to Europe the summer before that. It's made numerous trips to the East Coast. And it's become the bane of my existence.

Of all the people I know, I should have an Advance Directive. And it should be amazing. I would expect it to have rolled off my tongue without a moment's hesitation, curling toward the paper in a flurry of well-spoken dos and don'ts.

But I don't. And it's not that I haven't tried.

On its first trip, I completed part I before we reached 30,000 feet. The document asks for your designated power of attorney—in my case my husband, Mark, whose name and address I know quite well. But part II required heavy lifting. So I skipped ahead to parts III and IV. Organ donation? Check. Primary physician? Easy.

Four years later, part II remains incomplete.

This section is the crux of it all. It asks you to delineate your "instructions for health care." But it is so oversimplified that I am stumped and unable to go forward every time I look at it. You must choose between two checkboxes, A or B, and a few lines are provided below each for elaboration.

CHECKBOX A: CHOICE NOT TO PROLONG LIFE

I do not want my life to be prolonged if (1) I have an incurable and irreversible condition that will result in my death within a relatively short time, (2) I become unconscious and, to a reasonable degree of medical certainty, I will not regain consciousness, or (3) the likely risks and burdens of treatment would outweigh the expected benefits.

Okay, that feels clear enough. All of those conditions sound terrible to me. For me, an acceptable quality of life is about being able to engage in meaningful relationships with people, being able to talk, laugh, and connect. It is about not being lonely, confused, or scared. My grandmother lived for ten years with profound dementia; initially, she feigned recognition of her offspring but was unable in her final years even to recognize us. If I ever end up this way, I would want to be kept comfortable, to be treated with kindness, and when the time comes, to be allowed to die a natural death.

Similarly, I would not want a breathing tube thrust down my throat or to be the recipient of cardiac resuscitation if I am in the final stages of a terminal or life-limiting disease, even with all of my faculties present. I don't want to have my arms, legs, and airway tied to a bed for my final days or even weeks. I would not want large catheters threaded into my neck or groin to deliver dialysis if I were on the verge of death. These things happen all of the time, and I won't have it for myself.

But I am not currently in any of those conditions. So I read on.

CHECKBOX B: CHOICE TO PROLONG LIFE
I want my life to be prolonged as long as possible within the limits of generally accepted health care standards.

Of course I do. If there is a good chance that I will come back to my life. Even if I were a high-level quadriplegic like Christopher Reeve, who, despite his profound physical paralysis, was able to live an emotional and connected life at home with his family, I would welcome anything that the ICU had to offer to keep me going. If I were still able to hear my child laugh or understand a funny joke, I would fight the fight and accept all the consequences.

So which box is the right one for me to check? I don't know. My feelings are too complex, too nuanced, to fit into one little white square. If my family knows my general preferences, shouldn't they be able to drive the decisions accordingly? But then I start thinking about all of the times I have watched loving family members struggle to decide what is right for their loved one, even if they have previously discussed these topics. Prognostic uncertainty, difficulty getting clear information, and the anxiety and sadness of letting go—it can be profoundly difficult to know what to do. I want to provide my loved ones with more guidance than that. How will my husband and children, not medical people themselves, understand the details of my prognosis? What if it isn't yet perfectly clear to the doctors whether I will wake up again after a stroke? How long should they let the doctors keep trying? And what if I've already been attached to machines with a PEG and trach? When, and how, should they make the decision to disconnect those tubes and let me go?

There are good reasons I haven't yet filled out this form. On its own, it is far too simplistic to represent me. It would take a dissertation to elaborate on all of the possible decision points that may arise. And that dissertation feels like an attempt to control an event that is intrinsically uncontrollable.

Nonetheless, the fact remains that I am procrastinating on this. Intellectually, I know that I should complete the Advance Directive to the best of my ability and, even more important, go over its contents with my family. It can only be helpful to have another document clarifying my overall preferences, both as protection for me and as guidance for my family. I must not get lost in the technical complexity of the task. And I must push through the process despite the fact that thinking about my own death makes me profoundly sad. And feels so final.

chapter seven

The Personal Toll

A S A YOUNG INTERN with almost no experience, as I describe in Chapter One, I was able to mobilize an entire surgical unit in a sleeping hospital to manage my maternal grandmother's septic shock and save her life. Yet almost twenty years later, as a bona fide ICU and palliative care attending with a lot more confidence and know-how, I was unable to save my paternal grandmother from a frightening and uncomfortable death.

We all believed that after ten years of profound dementia my grandmother would want to die peacefully, without being attached to machines. We enrolled her in hospice, and she received wonderful care in her home. When she finally developed the aspiration-induced pneumonia so common to patients with end-stage dementia, she was admitted into the hospice facility for aggressive comfort management.

I flew to Montreal to be at her side. When I arrived, she was delirious and fighting to breathe. There was terror in her eyes and every breath was a struggle. A pulse oximeter next to her bed showed that her blood was only 79 percent oxygenated, a critically low reading. It was a Friday night and, in a bizarre déjà vu of my other grandmother's critical ordeal, only a bare-bones crew was staffing the facility. Where was the nurse? Why wasn't Grandma being given medication for her shortness of breath? Why wasn't her delirium being addressed? Why was a pulse oximeter on her finger at all when what mattered were her symptoms, not her numbers?

I snapped into action. This time, I wasn't trying to save a grandmother's life but rather to midwife her death. But I was unable to rally the troops. Years earlier, on my first tour of duty as an American doctor in a Canadian hospital, I had convinced nurses to start an IV and push two bags of saline into my grandmother before they could even reach the surgeon on call. But this time, I had to fight for a dose of morphine, even though it was already ordered in my paternal grandmother's chart to be given "as needed." I explained that I was a palliative care doctor, trained to work with opiates to mitigate symptoms. But the nurses were slow to respond and seemed to regard me with suspicion. When it was time for another dose, my request was followed by whispers at the nurses' station. It is a common myth that opioids shorten life in dying patients, and I was shocked to realize that these nurses thought I was trying to kill my grandmother.

The rest of the evening played out in a tug of war I found heartbreaking—the nurses clearly believed they were protecting their patient by withholding the morphine. My grandmother died the next morning, neither as calm nor as comfortable as she might have been.

It took some time for me to come to peace with this experience. In addition to watching my grandmother suffer unnecessarily, I was troubled by how the other health care workers had perceived me. They were suspicious of a physician who was not fighting to prolong her grandmother's life. It had been easier to mobilize the medical troops when I was rushing into an against-the-odds battle for life prolongation than when I was working to ease the inevitable. Saving the life of one grandmother connoted a type of heroism we can all understand. But in attempting to provide comfort during the last hours of my paternal grandmother's life, I was viewed as an antihero, someone to be regarded with suspicion, even outright hostility.

This experience, although a strikingly personal example, was emblematic of a phenomenon I encounter all too often in my work straddling these very different philosophies of care. And this clash of cultures, both in my environment and in my own psyche, has taken its toll.

Tattooed Tears

As I rounded the corner on my way to room 7, the nurse in charge of the patient in the adjacent room held his arms up, as if to prevent me from entering. "Dr. Zitter, we're okay in here. Really."

This was the punch line of a joke that I should have put a stop to days earlier.

During my past several stints attending in the ICU, I had noticed a few of the nurses chuckling every time a patient of mine was extubated, as if to imply that I extubated more than my share. In a way, it was true. ICU doctors aren't yet habituated to helping patients and families make decisions about the continued use of machines. I would often come onto service to find a number of dying patients on life support, many of their families unaware of the limited options before them. Therefore, my first few days on service often consisted of back-to-back family meetings and, frequently, at the families' request, the removal of life-prolonging machinery from one or more of my patients. Nonetheless, I feel compelled to add, the survival statistics for my patients have always matched those of my colleagues.

"No need for assistance," continued the nurse, grinning. "We're really okay." I looked at his arms, held out as if to protect his patient from me. There was the quality of an elementary school tease to the gesture, and I felt that protesting would only spur him on. I played cool, like you're taught to do with bullies on the playground. "You don't really feel that way," I said casually. "I know your type."

But the joke had taken on a life of its own. "You know those tattooed tears that gangsters get to mark their kills?" he said. "You could get a whole face full of them."

Now I stared at him, incredulous. I would deal with it later, in private. Besides, the family of my patient next door had seen me approaching and was waiting anxiously to continue our conversation. I turned around and stepped into room 7.

The patient was in a dense coma on top of multiple illnesses and dementia. He had suffered a cardiac arrest two weeks earlier and his brain had been irreversibly damaged due to inadequate oxygen. This man was unlikely ever to wake up again, and the time had come for his family to decide about a trach. During our meeting, it was decided that the patient would be extubated. As I walked out of the room, the same nurse, glancing at the medical student beside me, quipped, "You teaching that medical student how to kill too?"

He had gone way too far. "Don't you ever say anything like

that to me again," I said calmly. "It is unprofessional and unacceptable. And I don't think you really believe it." Around us stood the medical student, a respiratory therapist, and several other nurses. We walked away, and I could see my medical student was shaken. We had been working together all week, and he had repeatedly expressed interest in a patient-centered approach, arranging meetings with families, reading about prognoses, and struggling with the most important issues we deal with. He had joined me at every family meeting, even for patients he was not following.

"I can't believe he said that to you," he said.

I put my hand on his arm. "I'm sorry you saw that, but in a way, it's good. This is a reality you're going to face if you want to practice patient-centered medicine," I said. "Especially in an ICU."

Later that afternoon, as I was writing in a chart, the nurse found me. "I'm sorry I hurt your feelings," he said. "I was just joking." I nodded, and thanked him for the apology. I am confident he won't do that again, but his joke was a living example of what educational experts call "the hidden curriculum," an unofficial, unwritten syllabus that is shelved in medical education, in the ether of the clinical wards. Unlike the formal medical curriculum, which preaches professionalism in lecture halls and classrooms, this hidden curriculum teaches medical trainees by example. And data show that formal teachings are easily undermined by what happens in the real-life environment of patient care. Here, the pain and suffering of patients, as well as the clinicians who care for them, are more easily addressed through jokes or callous comments than honest acknowledgment of the pain. And even the most well-intentioned student can begin to mimic this defensive behavior, taking him a little further away from the patients he came to serve.

On a quiet Saturday in 2007, a colleague of mine was the critical care fellow on call at a VA hospital. Her census stood at eight seriously ill patients, most of them on ventilators. These patients were stable but critical—she had spent hours correcting their electrolytes, reviewing their antibiotics, and adjusting their ventilators—and she had finally found some time to sit and write her notes. The charge nurse that day was a weathered practitioner, a long-time ICU nurse. She approached my friend with a look of concern on her face. "You know that the patient in bed three's potassium has gotten critically high." My friend wasn't surprised. This patient had recently received chemotherapy for cancer, his fourth round, and had rapidly gone into septic shock. Now he was in the ICU with all organs failing on full machine support. As his kidney function plummeted, his ability to process potassium plummeted as well. And so the level of this electrolyte, dangerous in high quantities, was rising quickly. "Do you want to dialyze him?" the nurse asked my friend. And then she raised a skeptical eyebrow.

That raised eyebrow, my friend told me, was all she needed. Permission to question the paradigm. Dialysis would indeed reduce the potassium level, and when kidneys are failing, that is often considered the next logical step. But this patient was dying. Inserting a huge catheter at this point would not significantly delay the dying process, and it would certainly cause pain. Plus, it was dangerous—it could cause bleeding, infection, even pop the patient's lung. "Has anyone had a conversation with this family?" my friend asked. Nobody had. Nor, it turned out, had any of the families of the other four dying patients been informed of their dire conditions. And so my friend, with the support of the wise nurse, began to go bed by bed. She ended up calling in four of the families—to talk, to probe, to help them question. Each of these families was stunned, realizing that their loved ones were doing much more poorly than they had been led to believe. And so for each of those four patients, a decision was made to withdraw the breathing machine. They all died within twenty-four hours—naturally, without tubes in their mouths. My friend felt that she had achieved something significant. "Why haven't we had these conversations before?" she asked the nurse.

"That's just not the culture here," she was told.

But then one of the nurses in the unit grew alarmed over the number of extubations that day. She called the federal whistle-blower hotline for the VA. A government representative came to interview everyone in the ICU to determine if there had indeed been foul play, as was suggested. My friend was not interviewed, but her attending was. "Thanks to you, I was investigated," he said sternly—as though they had been looking into a crime rather than a vital health care decision. "You really should have called me before you extubated these people," he said. Looking back, my friend wishes she had done that. But she notes the fact that she would not have been expected to call him about other types of decisions, like intubating a patient or inserting a line. And she wonders whether, if she had called him that afternoon, he would have prevented her from doing what the patients' families requested her to do.

But the attending's body language, tone, and use of the word *investigation* made her think twice about whether she should be having these conversations so close together. In fact, whether she should be having them at all. Now, she told me, a decade later, she is just starting to gather her courage again to engage with patients and families in this way.

To me, this story illustrates in stark detail the pressures, particularly on ICU physicians, to keep treating dying patients until they die. If they aren't appearing to be struggling at all costs to keep a body alive for as long as technologically possible, they might be suspected of murdering their patients.

ICU Culture

The ICU is a tough place, and not only for its patients.

Despite the obvious difficulty of making often impossible decisions in quick succession, ICU culture is not designed to support reflective decision making. Its structure is hierarchical: all data and facts are presented to the attending physician, who then dispenses and oversees the plan for the day. Although there may be some back and forth, it is usually in the form of teaching. The students and residents generally take orders and do the attending's bidding. There is rarely room for the consideration of various approaches and the weighing of pros and cons. The ICU attending is expected to be calm and unruffled, making quick and definitive decisions like a general on a battlefield. The absence of these qualities can cause the troops to lose confidence, even trigger small acts of mutiny.

In contrast, during my palliative care rounds, input from everyone—the chaplain, the social worker, the medical student— is critical to my approach. Each possesses knowledge that I, as the physician, do not necessarily have. But when I try to bring this more collaborative style of decision making to ICU rounds, it can fall flat. This approach requires more rounding time, more reflection, more acknowledgment that there is not one right answer. And that is usually not what a stressed trainee or even a harried nurse seeks in her attending.

Of course, emergencies require definitive action. And such action must be guided by one leader, not a committee. But in truth, those moments of extreme urgency account for only a small percent of my time in the ICU. I have found that there is time in even the busiest of ICUs to bring attention to the complexity and human elements of most cases. If we don't strive to do that, then we risk making every ICU patient just a body to be kept alive.

In my early days of practicing these two seemingly disparate subspecialties, many doctors expressed surprise, even discomfort, at what they saw as a contradictory approach. "ICU and palliative care? Do those really go together?" was a common refrain. A family friend who was a well-respected chief of medicine at a Boston medical school once accused me of selling my patients a false bill of goods by incorporating palliative care techniques into my ICU toolbox, as if I was somehow less inclined to save their lives.

Many years ago, a colleague, while signing his patient out to me for the weekend, admonished me not to engage his almost-dead patient's family in a conversation about whether to keep him on the ventilator. "I've already kept him alive for six weeks," he said. "I can keep him going." It sounded to me almost as if he saw it as a sport. To give him the benefit of the doubt, he might have viewed this as his professional obligation. Yet this patient was so near death that his fragile lungs kept popping from the pressure of the breathing machine, prompting surgeons to insert plastic tubes through his chest into each new air pocket. The poor man looked like a hedgehog. Later that night, after another pop of the patient's lungs and stabilization, I couldn't stand it any longer. I sat with the worried family and told them of the patient's almost certain impending death. They listened in stunned silence and then asked me why they had not been told this before. "He's been suffering so much," they said. And there was no doubt, they told me, he would not have wanted this. "Take the tube out and let him go in peace," I was told. I'll never forget my colleague's expectant face on Monday morning as he gestured to me across the ICU. Thumbs up or thumbs down? Did you keep him alive or did you let him die?

At a case conference many years ago, my colleagues were debating, even conjuring, various last-ditch surgical and chemotherapeutic approaches to a patient with advanced brain cancer. I asked whether anyone had involved the patient in any of these conversations. I wondered aloud whether she might prefer to pursue a course of care focused on comfort management. Had anyone asked her what her preferences were? There were a few shrugs. Then one of my colleagues decided it was time to take a vote. "Okay," he said. "Who votes to do it Jessica's way, and do nothing?" I protested that I was not making recommendations one way or another about treatment, but simply advocating that we involve the patient in this conversation. My protests fell on deaf ears. I was viewed as defeatist.

Thankfully, these attitudes are beginning to shift. Both of these interactions happened many years ago. Change is definitely arriving, one person at a time, and I believe that someday soon it will be unacceptable to practice without considering the patient's needs above all else.

Yet we still have a ways to go. Recently, a colleague signed patients out to me with a sigh of relief, saying, "So glad you're coming on. Half of our patients could really use a palliative touch." While I am glad that the culture is becoming more receptive to these practices, I still look forward to the day when all ICU physicians are comfortable with, trained in, and highly proactive about engaging patients and families on these difficult topics. A day when interventions such as end-of-life conversations and writing orders to allow a natural death are perceived as expanding options, rather than limiting them. We aren't there yet, but I believe the tide is beginning to shift.

Increasing attention is being paid to the phenomenon of physician burnout, characterized by emotional exhaustion and a lack of enthusiasm for work. It has been found to be alarmingly prevalent in doctors compared to the general population. Its impacts, which include high rates of depression and compassion fatigue, are severe for both the doctor and her patients.

I understand firsthand why this might be. Most doctors I know are well-intentioned, compassionate, and hardworking people. And we have taken on the almost Sisyphean task of addressing illness and suffering. Frequent exposure to stress, grief, and death are a daily part of the job. And most physicians are subject to frustrating bureaucratic hurdles on top of that. But the discouragement or burnout that I have experienced as a palliative care physician is in its own category altogether.

Anecdotal evidence I have gathered from palliative care friends and colleagues around the country affirms my belief that we are at particular risk of burnout relative to the rest of the medical profession. And we all agree that this is not caused simply by witnessing more death and dying than other specialties.

The subspecialty of palliative care medicine is relatively new in the history of modern medicine. All new things take time to become accepted and integrated into routine practice. Before the advent of our modern technologies, these skills were part of the general practice of medicine. But after being rendered obsolete beginning in the mid-twentieth century, doctors grew accustomed to practicing without them.

Ironically, although many of these skills are as old as the hills, reintroducing them has proven difficult. Financial compensation rates are a reflection of perceived value. Palliative care is one of the lowest-paid specialties, with a median compensation of

$215,000 per year, while a dermatologist who performs special-ized skin cancer surgery makes over $700,000. The implication being that our skills are ancillary. It's hard not to internalize this on some level.

From what I've seen, other physicians may feel that our presence is unnecessary, possibly even threatening. Our input regarding patient-centered decision making and goal setting is something doctors tend to believe they are already doing, or at least should be doing, themselves.

The palliative care physicians I have spoken with also note that at times other doctors perceive them as a threat to their pa-tients; each had examples mirroring my experience with the sur-geon in Chapter Four, who fired me from the case because she believed I would drain her patient of hope. Because we acknowl-edge death, other physicians may see us as defeatist. We have all had the experience of being asked by the team to "keep the con-sult focused on symptoms" as opposed to discussing bad news and assessing goals of care. They worry we will sap their patients' will to live.

The fact that we are consultants, and not the primary "own-ers" of the patient adds another layer of complexity to our mission. I have myself acted as a consultant in three different capacities— as a pulmonologist, an intensivist, and a palliative care doctor— and I am struck by the difference in how I am commonly treated in these roles. In the first two, my word feels like gospel. "How many milligrams of prednisone should we start? What studies should I send the lavage specimen for?" But when my palliative care input is requested, I am sometimes instructed on which areas are permissible and which are off-limits. "Please deal only with his pain issues. Don't talk about the breathing machine. We're still waiting to hear back from the oncologists so please don't talk about chemotherapy with the patient—we want the oncologist to do that. And definitely don't bring up hospice." And we must display good consultation etiquette in order to keep the consults coming. Often palliative care teams feel as if they are on constant trial to gain acceptance and consultations.

The acknowledgment of the unique stressors of palliative care physicians is a very recent phenomenon. Given how small and crucial this community is, I feel we must do everything possible to prevent any losses, whether in body or spirit, of its members. We will all stand to benefit.

Moral Distress

It was 12:05 P.M. at the monthly meeting of the ethics committee. Everyone had a sandwich, a bag of chips, and a bottle of water. The chair picked up the stapled handout of last week's minutes and whipped through them. "Move to approve?"

Several people murmured, "Approved."

"Second?"

Someone raised his hand in affirmation.

"Does anyone have new business? New cases?"

Her co-chair raised his hand. "There's a case from a satellite hospital that we've been asked to look at."

A few people sighed. Our hospital alone provided us with a full list of cases. We didn't have much bandwidth for those from outside.

"I'm not really sure what they're asking for here," he said. "Seems pretty straightforward." The co-chair went on to describe the case. An elderly man with profound dementia on a ventilator in their ICU. He had been continuously aspirating food and it seemed to the doctors he would only continue to worsen. He was agitated, disoriented, and uncomfortable, and the doctors were very distressed at the instructions they had been given by the legal surrogate. Keep him alive at all costs, she said.

The patient's long-time girlfriend was the surrogate. The notarized Advance Directive left no question that the patient had intended for her to make medical decisions on his behalf. All other family members were long estranged. And the woman seemed to know the patient's values and preferences; he had told her repeatedly over the many years they'd been together, she said, that he would want to be kept alive as long as possible if it ever came to that. Well, it had, and here we were.

As the committee began to discuss the case, several people stated they could not see any ethical conflict. We had a legal surrogate enacting substituted judgment based on actual conversations she had with the patient. By the letter of the law, as well as the code of medical ethics as it stands, we had all we needed to render an opinion and sign off the case. "Shall we move on?" the co-chair asked.

I shook my head. Something wasn't sitting right with me. The case was striking a very familiar chord. I saw that we probably weren't going to help these doctors at all. The help they needed, I realized, did not fall under the official jurisdiction of the ethics committee. The committee's charge is primarily to promote patients' rights by examining all angles of the complex, usually conflict-laden cases brought before it. They must consider not only ethical aspects, but legal ones as well. And since, as we have seen, there are often more questions than answers, ethics committees' recommendations often involve seeking more information and understanding. But these physicians had reached out because, although this case met all legal and ethical requirements, they were highly uncomfortable with what they were being asked to do.

They needed moral, not ethical, support.

Although I didn't know these doctors personally, I knew first-hand the feeling that must have propelled them to bring this case to our committee. I knew they had better things to do than to collect and organize the necessary documentation. This was work they had done on their own time.

I thought of the many times I had brought similar cases to the committee, and walked away with a sense of frustration. I'd come to the ethics committee with these cases because I had exhausted all other avenues for consultation—colleagues, the palliative care team, even the legal department. But none of their suggestions had helped, and I came hoping to find some sort of moral support to carry on.

The concept of moral distress was first defined by Andrew Jameton in the nursing literature in 1984. It has gained traction over the past several years, and the medical community has slowly followed nursing in acknowledging its existence. Jameton described moral distress as a "perceived violation of one's core values and duties," and it is now seen as responsible for major problems among health care providers, including feelings of guilt, anger, and self-blame, as well as anxiety and depression. Some physicians quit the profession entirely. And for those who stay, this suffering cannot help but affect vulnerable patients, as burn-out and compassion fatigue have also been attributed to moral distress.

It makes sense to me that the phenomenon was first noticed by nurses. They are professionally bound to follow orders from physicians with whom they may disagree. And they are, in a sense, more "in the trenches" with the patients than are we physicians, who can breeze through rooms and busy ourselves with our procedures. And so nurses witness more of the suffering yet have less control over it. Nor do they have the same technologies and procedures to distract them that we doctors do.

By my read of the literature as well as from my own experience, a hefty portion of this moral distress occurs when health care providers feel they are prolonging lives that shouldn't be prolonged. And in doing so, they often follow orders that were written by their own hands. Mildred Solomon and her colleagues showed that a majority (80 percent) of twenty-five neonatal ICU physicians agreed with this statement: "Sometimes I feel we are saving children who shouldn't be saved." In contrast, only a minority (8 percent) agreed with this statement: "Sometimes I feel we give up on children too soon."

Yet it's not that simple. There have been many instances when I have worked to prolong the life of an obviously dying person with no moral distress at all. The difference is that these are cases in which I feel confident the patient or surrogate has truly understood the realities and possible burdens of the requested treatments. There has been a meaningful transaction of information, from my honest breaking of bad news to a full description of the potential burdens of the treatment options. If I am confident that a patient or his surrogate has assimilated the possible outcomes of prolonged life support—the repeated admissions for septic shock, sacral decubitus ulcers, loneliness, custodial dehumanization— then I can bear to keep the patient alive. While it might be painful to witness, I don't feel moral distress. If I had had the opportunity to really talk to Uncle Barry or Vincent about their preferences, I do not believe I would have experienced the moral distress I did when watching them suffer through their final weeks.

My worry, at the risk of sounding paternalistic, is that people who request this treatment rarely understand the realities involved in "doing everything." And the reasons for this frequently are out of my control. While we've seen that we doctors don't always explain it very well, often it is the patient or family members who turn a deaf ear, even if we try.

So as the committee chair was preparing to move us on to the next case, I raised my hand. "I think these doctors are asking for something else from us," I said. As I continued talking, another clinician began to nod her head. She had felt the same sense of frustration, she told us, when she had brought one of her cases to the committee the previous year. She had left the meeting having heard a lot of opinions and suggestions but carrying the same feelings of muted despair that compelled her to bring the case forward in the first place.

As we continued our discussion, it became clear that doctors, whether members of the committee or not, needed support for their moral distress. And in most systems there is no institutional place to find that support. Some hospitals have begun to address this need with events like Schwartz Center Rounds, in which caregivers discuss patient cases from an emotional vantage point. But if we expect health care providers to do the hard work of patient-centered care, we must provide them with more space and support for their moral distress. Otherwise, it is not only us but our patients who will suffer.

Too Late to Talk

Around five years ago I treated a patient with a secret he'd been keeping for years.

When I met him, he was breathing as if through a narrow straw. His lungs, pulpy and inflamed on the chest X-ray, were in no shape to filter oxygen. He grabbed at my arms like a drowning man as I tried to refit the BiPAP mask on his face.

Do something, screamed his eyes.

EXTREME MEASURES

You bet I will, said mine.

Mr. Williams was a forty-nine-year-old man with pneumocystis pneumonia (PCP), a pneumonia of advanced AIDS. For reasons he would carry to his grave, he had declined to take the miraculous anti-HIV medications offered to him five years earlier. These likely would have changed his prognosis from a few years to a lifetime of chronic but manageable illness. It may have been denial; it may have been shame. This man had told nobody he was sick and admonished me to make sure no one found out, including his mother, who was waiting nervously in the lobby. He'd been in the emergency room for shortness of breath the previous month but had left AMA—against medical advice—after we'd arranged for him to be admitted. He'd been given pills for his pneumonia but evidently hadn't taken many of them.

And now he was making what was probably his final landing in the ICU at the inner-city hospital where I worked. He was clearly dying.

I huddled outside his room with my team to discuss our next steps. We would, of course, intubate him. That's why we had been called. But I was quite confident it wouldn't help. Having done my residency and fellowship in inner-city hospitals in the early 1990s, before the use of antiretroviral medications, I knew that by the time intubation was required for PCP, patients were almost surely beyond saving. When intubated, they almost always died tethered to their breathing machines.

I was in a quandary. This was a man who had chosen, when he was capable of choosing, to resist medical interventions. Yet at his most vulnerable moment, I was about to attach him to a breathing machine. He was dying rapidly, and yet the things that I was trained to do probably wouldn't work—and he probably didn't want them. But I couldn't know that for sure. Was it my place to decide to pass up on a chance to prolong his life, vanishingly slim though it may be? We couldn't talk to his mother about his AIDS and explain why intubating him probably wouldn't help. We couldn't tell her about his refusal of medical treatments or his avoidance of the hospital. Our hands were tied from using her as a surrogate. And there wasn't anyone else to talk to. No children, no siblings. What about the patient himself? He was still alert, still nodding and shaking his head appropriately to questions. But he was struggling. Breathing took every ounce of his energy. And he was scared, with wide and terrified eyes. How could I stress him further? Yet who else was there to ask?

I decided to talk to him.

But when I walked into the room, I lost my resolve. The mask was tight over his face, cutting into the bridge of his nose; his mouth sucked desperately at the air. He was leaning forward in the bed, trying to expand his rib cage. He had to be breathing fifty times a minute. It was painful to watch. I walked back out of the room to collect myself. I stood there, frozen in doubt, until one of my medical students saw me. You have to talk to him, she said. I knew she was right—so I walked back into the room.

By this time, the drugs for intubation were being drawn up. The respiratory therapist had wheeled the ventilator into the room. Students and residents were collecting in the hallways, as they do when any procedure is about to be performed. Often with emergency intubations, patients aren't aware of what is happening around them. But this patient was; he had noticed the activity and it was clear his anxiety level was rising. This man needed the chance to opt out.

I approached the bed and gently laid my hand over his, which was gripping the bed rail. "I just want to check with you before we do what we usually do when someone is having problems breathing," I said. "I'm very concerned that this breathing tube, if we put it in, will never come out. That you'll die on the ventilator. You'll never eat again. Never drink again."

He stared at me, gasping like a drowning man. I couldn't read his emotions at all. He wasn't capable of a conversation, and so I had to ask him a yes or no question. "Would it be okay with you to stay attached to this machine until you die?" It was the best I could summon in the few seconds that I had.

He stared at me. Then he moved his head in a way that resembled a nod. It was the closest I could get to an answer. We had no time. We put the tube in.

The patient lived for a few hours on the ventilator, before his blood pressure collapsed and he died. I was in my car driving home when my pager went off, signaling a Code Blue. I knew without looking that it was in his room.

The next morning I debriefed with my team. These conversations usually entail Monday-morning quarterbacking of the code, deconstructing our efforts in the context of the patient's physiological deterioration. But I was most interested in my team's emotional experience. Watching and participating in a grueling death is traumatizing, but doctors are expected to somehow deal with it and move on. I've learned about the importance of an emotional debrief from the palliative care community, and now I can't imagine how we expect our young trainees to progress through their training in a healthy and productive way without it.

The medical student said she would never forget it. The intern said, "No offense, Dr. Zitter, but I'm uncomfortable that the last thing the patient heard was that he was probably going to die." My heart lurched in my chest. That had been my worst fear—that I was inflicting more suffering on the patient by trying to get to the truth. I asked the intern if he would have preferred that we had just gone forward and intubated without talking to the patient. What if the patient would have chosen to opt out? He didn't have an answer.

These decisions are difficult in any case, but with secrecy, physical distress, and an unclear set of personal preferences, there is no real way to know what to do in the very few moments that are left. All options available to me felt brutal. Trying to talk to a dying man in extremis about his mortality. Not trying to talk to a dying man in extremis about his mortality. What would you do?

I will never know if my attempts to determine and honor his preferences ended up making things worse. I will never know if intubating him brought even more suffering to the final moments of his life. I suspect both are true—that despite my best intentions, I caused this man added layers of distress before he died. Every split-second decision has the potential to make things better—or significantly worse. That is a lot to live with.

Friend or Consultant

I was cooking dinner a few years ago when I received a text from my friend Alan: "Wld u speak to Jen's frnd who's dying?" Before I had a chance to put down my spoon, my phone rang. Alan went on without a beat. "She's talking about having more chemotherapy but she weighs ninety-eight pounds and can barely walk. Her doctor wants to do it. We think it's a terrible idea. Can you talk to her?"

Then Alan and Jennifer took turns explaining. Their friend had been diagnosed with cancer years ago and had tried every treatment under the sun. She was a single parent with a young daughter. Her status had worsened precipitously over the past few weeks, and now it seemed she was nearing the end of her life. Jennifer had been with her friend in the oncology suite when the doctor told her that there were no more treatment options. But her friend refused to accept this news. She would go to a specialized cancer treatment center, she told Jennifer, or maybe to Mexico. Hospice was completely out of the question. She wasn't ready to give up.

Listening to them, I felt torn. If I called Jennifer's friend, I might help her understand that more treatment would almost definitely not help and could even shorten her life. A recent study in *JAMA Oncology* showed that even active patients with metastatic cancer were apt to have a significant worsening of quality of life from chemotherapy, without extension of life. Hospice, on the other hand, could help on both counts—quality, certainly, and maybe even quantity. Shouldn't I try to explain this to her?

I should, I knew. But it was three days before my daughter's bat mitzvah. People were arriving from the East Coast tomorrow. We still had alterations to do, welcome bags to fill, a music playlist to compile. I was getting phone calls from friends and relatives every hour with urgent questions or requests. My daughter was nervous and needed my support. And while this conversation might be quick, it would more likely be long and emotional, maybe requiring a series of follow-up calls. I was completely torn. I had never before refused a request to walk someone through the dying process, no matter from whom—friend, family, vague acquaintance. I sometimes spent many hours over multiple days on the phone with unknown physicians at the request of patients and their loved ones. I felt I had no choice, given how few resources there were for families whose doctors were failing them. At my fiftieth birthday party, six of the toasts came from friends thanking me for providing them with this kind of support. And refusing now, in favor of a celebration, felt awful.

On the other end of the line, Alan waited for my reply. I steeled myself, and then I said no. I couldn't stop apologizing, and I have continued to do so long after the woman's death. It was a bad one, and I will never know if I could have changed its course. But I was at my limit, nearing overwhelm; I felt I had no more to give.

There's a flip side to this coin, too. I have many friends who have turned to me as an adviser and gotten more than they bargained for. A few years ago, the father of one of my closest friends began to die. This was evident to me from the medical details she shared. But the family and medical team were still pursuing an aggressive treatment plan, and I worried that the suffering was outweighing the benefit. She would call me with good news from specialists that really wasn't good news at all. The team had found that he was carrying a virus, she told me one day. They would try to treat it, which seemed to her like a step in the right direction. But I knew it wouldn't change the outcome. He had lymphoma everywhere. In his brain, his abdomen. Treating a virus wouldn't turn this train around. And it would prevent him from coming home, which he had been asking to do for weeks. I strongly encouraged her to bring him home on hospice. That never happened.

At a certain point I began to worry that my input was upsetting her. I suspected she was avoiding my phone calls. Although my friend denied it, I worried that my attempts to deliver the truth felt unsupportive, possibly even cruel. And while our friendship is as strong as ever, I wonder sometimes if instead of trying to educate her, I should have just been a sympathetic friend.

Too Many Possibilities

In straddling the disparate worlds of the ICU and palliative care, I reap the benefits of a broader set of skills and offerings, but also the challenges of merging two medical perspectives. Some of these are simply logistical. Given that I alternate between these two very different roles, colleagues sometimes wonder which hat I'm wearing on a particular day. "Are you on palliative or ICU?" they ask me, expecting a completely different set of behaviors depending on the whims of that month's schedule. Often I take care of the same patient in different capacities. I might end the week as the ICU attending only to come back on Monday on the palliative care service, consulting on many of the patients I referred the week before. Other weeks I enter the ICU to attend on patients whom I had followed on the palliative care consult team the week prior.

But other challenges in merging these worlds are emotional, even spiritual. As my training and experience have broadened in both these worlds, my mission has grown murkier and I have paradoxically grown less convinced that there are always clear answers. If I am expert at anything, it is at navigating uncertainty, facing self-doubt, accepting that there are no easy answers. I cannot pursue my ICU instincts without seriously weighing my palliative care ones, and vice versa. I cannot assume that the way I treated one patient is the way I should treat another. I cannot assume that what is an acceptable functional state for one person is right for another. I have come to see that there are no clear blueprints to follow. And this can be a difficult place to practice. It can be draining, and tremendously lonely. Yet I see on the horizon signs of hope. I see the public beginning to ask for care that will better serve its needs. I see colleagues beginning to seek training in skills, like communication, that used to be considered ancillary. I look forward to the day when death is considered a part of life, when our health care system is agile and sophisticated enough to recognize the dying process and refrain from medicalizing it. I long, too, for the day when we health care providers are better supported to give that care.

chapter eight

Sharing the Journey

I N JUNE 2014 *The New York Times Magazine* published an essay on training firefighters titled "Baptism by Fire." The writer, N. R. Kleinfield, told the story of Jordan Sullivan, a probationary fire officer, or "probie," at his first fire. The piece was gorgeous, filled with glossy pictures of firefighters in regalia looking modest yet heroic.

I was struck by the similarities between firefighting and my own career.

Jordan Sullivan was ninety-six days into his probationary training before he ever experienced a fire. Just as I awaited my first medical code as an intern, Jordan itched for his turn to join the fight. Much as I had been inspired to join the medical profession by the hero doctors who had gone before me, Sullivan was inspired to become a firefighter by the courageous acts of the New York firefighters following 9/11.

Jordan Sullivan's first fire went extremely well. Nobody died. No one even got seriously injured. And Sullivan was the most heroic of all; he "made a grab," saving the life of a baby. It was almost unheard of for a probie to make a grab; some of the elite in his unit had made only one or two grabs in their entire careers.

In fighting fire, the stakes are high and the rewards great. Seconds count, and therefore the organization is almost military, with clear hierarchies and protocols demanding lightning-quick action. On arrival at the scene of the fire, Jordan's chief surveyed the location and strategized his approach within minutes. One stairwell in the building was designated the "attack" stairs; the other was reserved for evacuation of residents. The team worked together like a well-oiled machine, with clear orders issued to each member from the chief on his handheld unit. Everyone knew his place and his job—Hayden assessed the perimeter, Kehoe proceeded to the roof to open the doors, and Sullivan, Crowley, and LaBarbera were dispatched to find the fire and look for victims.

I began to think of how we assign roles during a code. The person "running" the code surveys the patient's condition and devises a plan of attack. She then assigns other members to their jobs: one on the chest to start compressions, another to thread a central line into a large vessel, and a third to record every drug and event that occurs. The code follows one of several carefully scripted protocols based on the etiology of the cardiac or pulmonary arrest.

But that, I realized, is where the similarities end. A firefighter has a very specific and appropriate charge: to save any lives he can. There is little reflection required. Just get the person out. What came before or happens down the line are not part of the equation. But this is not the case for a doctor, even one in the business of saving lives.

There are clearly situations in medicine where swift and definitive action must be taken to save a life. And in those moments we doctors must go into full battle against death, much as firefighters do. But once the crisis has passed, or, better yet, before it happens at all, it is the doctor's responsibility to find out if the patient wants to be a part of that battle. And subsequent decisions must be thoughtfully crafted with input from the patient, or at least his surrogate. Here I know of no simple protocols, no rapid-fire steps to take. But I do know that instead of leading the fight against the disease in our patients, we must now be beside them, sitting on their beds, holding their hands, asking questions, and listening intently. Action must now derive from human connection and the interchange of information about how the patient wants to live. Or die. While I may be the expert on the patient's disease, I am not the expert on the patient.

In my opinion, this critical post-crisis work cannot be carried out by a medical team working in the hierarchical firefighting mode, where one chief calls out orders for others to obey without reflection or discussion. That model is not conducive to patient-centered decision making, which requires the gathering of all possible information and the consideration of all perspectives.

How might we foster a team structure that is better able to serve the patient after the crisis has been averted? Thinking back over the hundreds, if not thousands, of medical teams in which I have participated over the years, I recognize certain patterns. Some of these have felt healthy, others less so. Each team is like a transient family in which members must work together to get a very stressful job done. An attending leader and a sprinkling of residents and medical students are randomly thrown together for several weeks at a time. Each team quickly develops its own organic microculture, and the departure or addition of even one member can change the entire group dynamic. Even as the attending physician, I do not have complete control over the dynamic of my team. One week I may find myself with a collaborative group that is eager to reflect on our approach to both the medical and non-medical aspects of the case. The next week, such discussions may fall flat and go nowhere.

In 2013 I attended a lecture sponsored by the American Academy of Hospice and Palliative Care Medicine. A social worker in the department of pain medicine and palliative care at The Mount Sinai Hospital in New York, Terry Altilio, gave a talk titled "Team Process and Communication." She described the factors that make for an effective and healthy medical team, one that will likely be more successful in delivering patient-centered care.

She began by describing some of the many factors that might impede group function, including clashes of personalities, belief systems, or philosophies of care. The culture of the hospital or institution can play a significant role as well. How hierarchical is the environment? Does the attending encourage collaborative input or instead make pronouncements about next steps? How does the group deal with uncertainty? Is anyone willing to ask the unasked questions?

While there is no changing the personalities and histories that each of us brings to the group, Terry Altilio described how a positive team dynamic can be cultivated with intention. It usually needs to come from the top, she said, from the attendings and senior residents. There are strategies for fostering an environment that encourages people to express their feelings and question the plan of care without fear of judgment. Time can be set aside on rounds for reflection and deliberation of complex cases. The voicing of moral distress can be encouraged. And there can be general acknowledgment of the presence of complexity and nuance instead of searching for that one right answer.

I recently watched as one of my attending colleagues, in an attempt to solicit input from his team on the prognosis of a very sick patient, ripped a sheet of paper into eight pieces and held a secret ballot. Every member indicated anonymously that he believed the patient would die during this hospitalization, although none had felt comfortable verbalizing this sentiment. Now out in the open, the team was able to put the emperor's clothes back on and make an honest assessment of which treatments would be of actual benefit to the patient. I thought this was an ingenious technique.

Still, I long for the day when open and honest discussion does not require the use of a secret ballot. I believe this will require structural changes in our rounding procedures, as well as a continued shift in our culture. Collaboration and reflection should be part of the care of every single patient. Once the fire is out, the team must be equipped to do the other, more difficult work of attending to the patient.

Caring Together

A few years ago I gave a lecture at a local hospital. One of the interventional cardiologists described his approach to patients with cardiogenic shock, for whom the prognosis for survival is in the 40 percent range. He acknowledged that decision making was very difficult for the family in these cases—and for the team as well. "You have to make a decision with the family," he said. "If they say they're all in, you just need to go for it."

Yet he admitted that shifting goals of care was not his forte. Many of his patients who didn't do well remained on maximal life support until they died in the cardiac ICU. But he didn't think it was right; he was searching for something different.

Then he suggested something that sounded new to me. In

cases like these, he asked, with an unclear trajectory, couldn't a team approach to care be in place right from the start? Listening to him, I realized he was asking for help. If a palliative care clinician was involved right from the start, he continued, ongoing communication would come from a more neutral clinician, not one caught up in the "go for it" effort. This arrangement would allow the cardiologists to focus on their procedure while family members would be provided with realistic information at each new development, allowing them to continuously reassess the care plan. A palliative care doctor could support all members of the team: the family, the interventional doctors, and, most important, the patient.

I thought this was a brilliant idea. A stepping stone on the path toward culture change. With communication support embedded in his service, the interventional cardiologist might become more comfortable integrating these skills and techniques into his own practice. And then teaching them to his trainees and co-workers.

Even those doctors most competent in their chosen field might need a guiding hand here.

Heroic Doctors Ask for Help

It was a Monday morning on the palliative care service, and I was responding to pages regarding consults that had accumulated over the weekend. The first concerned a sixty-five-year-old man with metastatic prostate cancer. He had been diagnosed with the aggressive cancer six months earlier. He had continued to decline and his fiancée felt she could no longer care for him at home, so he was sent to a nursing home. He was admitted to our ICU a month before I met him, with septic shock from a urinary infection. Although his blood pressure had improved with aggressive treatment, he remained in the ICU, suffering complication after complication—first a blood clot in the leg released into his lungs, and then a dangerous stomach bleed due to the blood-thinning medications treating the clot. A few days before I finally met him, he had begun to breathe more shallowly, with a resultant rise in his blood carbon dioxide levels. This phenomenon causes a narcotic-like haze. The ICU doctors were considering whether to re-intubate him.

The doctor who had requested my consultation is someone I respect very much. A former chief resident, he was at this point in his third year on staff as a hospitalist attending. The care he provided to his patients was always thoughtful and thorough. He had excellent technical skills, was a sharp diagnostician, and radiated kindness.

As he described the case over the phone, I heard his distress. He had spent a lot of time with this patient over the previous week, managing his medical ups and downs. Although the doctor didn't say it outright, I could tell he believed the patient was dying. Weeks earlier, he had talked to the man about his preferences and learned his patient did not want to undergo intubation or cardiac resuscitation. I listened as my colleague struggled with what to do next.

"I performed an ultrasound of his chest," he said, "to see if he had a pleural fluid that I could tap off to improve his breathing. I didn't see anything, but maybe I should get a CT scan to get a better view."

I recognized his conundrum. It was one with which I was very familiar: feeling sure that a patient was dying, but not feeling able to stop trying to prevent it. We agreed to meet at the patient's room in an hour, after I had examined him.

After reading the chart and examining the patient, I was confident that my colleague's instincts were correct. The likelihood that this patient had any reversible cause of his deterioration was so low as to make further diagnostic or therapeutic interventions more risky than beneficial. His body was shutting down.

My hospitalist colleague entered the ICU as I was writing my note. "I agree with you," I said. "I don't think we can turn this around." He nodded vigorously. "That's what I thought you'd say." We agreed that it was time to focus on aggressive symptom management and pursue comfort measures only. We started a low-dose opioid patch to manage the pain from the ulcers on the patient's back, which had been the most troublesome symptom.

We made the patient DNR/DNI as he had requested, but we didn't even have time to start pain management. Within twenty minutes of my leaving the ICU, he died. It was peaceful, I was told by the nurse.

I don't believe my value to this case derived from my training in palliative care or from my expertise in pulmonary and ICU medicine. What I offered here was support for an excellent doctor to do what he ultimately knew was the right thing to do, even though everything in his training conspired against it. Had I been in his place, I would have benefited from someone acting in my role. Together, we helped each other honor the patient's stated goals of care.

I received three other consults that Monday, and every one of those was essentially for moral support as well. Support for the medical team to recommend to the patient's family a change of course from continued treatment to palliation.

I believe that no doctor should have to stand alone in making life or death decisions. In our current medical culture, one doctor makes most of the decisions for a given patient during a particular hospitalization. But this, I believe, can simply be too much moral responsibility for one human being to hold. Sharing impressions and processing a case with a colleague gives a doctor more confidence to broaden the range of options beyond the single-minded pursuit of life prolongation.

Currently, there is no easy mechanism for doing this. One can request a formal palliative care consult, as my colleague did, but this requires an investment of time and a good dose of humility, as many requesting doctors feel that they should be able to make these decisions on their own. Alternatively, we doctors may bounce the occasional case off each other in the halls—if we happen to pass the right person at the right time in the right hallway. But these chance meetings are random and fleeting, lacking the time and space for us to reliably engage in this critical support. I believe medicine needs a mechanism enabling doctors managing dying patients to get this kind of collegial support. Even the best of doctors will be the better for it.

The Art of De-escalation

I remember recommending to my residents that we stop testing blood from an arterial line in a patient who would likely die within hours. Her family was prepared and standing vigil. We had done everything we could do to turn things around, but the patient was rapidly worsening. "It's not going to hurt her because she already has a line in place," one of them said. Yet the information wouldn't change our management. It most likely wouldn't hurt the patient, I conceded, but I was trying to teach my residents that the philosophy of doing more was misguided at this point. This was a moment, I explained, to usher in a very different paradigm of care. Thus I held firm.

I found out in the end someone had ordered the test anyway.

Not only do doctors need support when it comes to the *whether* and *when* of shifting goals, they also need the skills to implement the *how.*

We have innumerable protocols for *doing* things to patients but almost none for *undoing* things to them. When goals of care are downshifted to focus on comfort, we are still left to figure out how to do it. While there is a standard protocol for managing septic shock or a heart attack, allowing someone to have a natural death can be elusive.

There is some precedent for lowering the intensity of care in the field of infectious disease medicine. Early in the course of a severe infection, before the species of bacteria has been identified under the microscope, doctors prescribe many different classes of antibiotics simultaneously. This is referred to as a shotgun approach, and it is an attempt to gain control of the infection before it overtakes the patient. But as soon as there is more information about the exact type of bacteria present, we doctors rapidly reduce the number of antibiotics to the one or maybe two that are needed. This is called *de-escalation* of antibiotic therapy.

I believe we need de-escalation protocols for those patients at the end of life who do not desire continued life-prolonging treatment. Right now, we wing it. It is as if we are forging a new path each time, with all of the resultant conflict that comes with matters of life and death, both within ourselves and among the team.

Some ICUs have protocols for de-escalating certain types of treatment, such as withdrawing a ventilator from a dying patient. But I have not personally seen any other de-escalation protocols in use. While removing a breathing tube is one thing, turning the dial down on blood pressure support medication (pressors) is another. In the first case, you're removing a highly uncomfortable, extremely invasive object—one that has been sitting at the core of the patient's body. Removing it usually brings visible relief, if not to the patient, then to her family. But decreasing the drip rate on pressors is a different matter altogether. These do not appear invasive or uncomfortable; they enter the body through IV tubing tucked behind the patient. But they do have risks, including increasing the potential for fatal heart arrhythmias and decreasing blood flow to fingers and toes, which can cause a gangrenelike condition. And more to the point, these medications, like the breathing machine, are possibly keeping the person alive when his body is trying to die.

And there are other big questions. Do we continue the dialysis? What about antibiotics? What about artificial nutrition through the feeding tube? When fed, a body might be kept alive for many years—and this should be a consideration if the goal of care is allowing a natural death. All of these treatments carry risk and no significant benefit for a dying patient. And yet it can be emotionally challenging for the doctor to remove them, one after the other. A protocol can help.

Of course, not all protocols will work for all patients. A patient who is hoping to see a loved one from out of state one last time before he dies might choose to continue blood pressure support medications even though he wants the breathing tube removed. Another patient may benefit from ongoing antibiotic treatment for an infection that is causing pain. But protocols can still be helpful here. Used as a guide, their very existence can serve to encourage more conversation about how exactly the patient wants to be treated, right up to the end.

Each case is unique. But most of the time, when the goal is to allow a natural death, we must have an approach to withdraw the many treatments that have been attached to the patient in order to keep her alive.

Steven Cook, a morbidly obese man in his fifties, had been admitted to our hospital floor with respiratory distress resulting from a combination of pneumonia and sleep apnea. The moment he arrived in the emergency room, he was fitted with a BiPAP mask. Then fluids and antibiotics were started. He remained on the medical floor for a few weeks, his illness at a slow rumble, not significantly worsening but not getting better either. Every time he stopped using the BiPAP for any significant time, he quickly tired out and required the mask's support again. A few weeks into his admission, he developed an ulcer in his colon that began to bleed briskly. He was rushed to the operating room where he was quickly intubated and underwent the removal of half of his colon. He was then sent to the ICU to recover. But when I first met him two weeks later, he was still attached to life support. The blood loss from his hemorrhaging ulcer, although long since replenished, had seriously damaged his kidneys and possibly his brain. His kidney dysfunction might eventually necessitate dialysis treatment three times per week, a quality of life hit for many, but a way to stay alive. However, there is no treatment available for a brain that has been permanently damaged by lack of blood supply, and it would take weeks to determine if this was the case.

When I took over his care, he remained completely dependent on the breathing machine, despite the resolution of his pneumonia. He was only lightly sedated but completely unresponsive. His intestinal bleed had been cured by the surgery, and his shock resolved, but he was not bouncing back. His kidneys were failing, his neurologic prognosis unclear, and he was barely breathing on his own. And now we were at the two-week trach point.

I was called in as the palliative care consultant to help the busy

ICU team assess goals of care with the family. Even though this man was relatively young, the team had become concerned that the patient would not improve.

Steven's daughter and son-in-law seemed to understand the basics—the breathing disturbance, the stomach bleed—but they didn't know that the team was concerned about the bigger picture. That he might never get better. And now, I explained, the time had come for us to decide whether to trach him and keep going or to consider switching goals of care from cure to comfort. He might be dying, I told them.

They looked at me in surprise. They had followed the team's ministrations carefully. As each of Steven's medical problems cropped up, they had conferred with the team on the plans of attack. True, they would have expected improvement by now, but they hadn't allowed negative thoughts to enter their minds, choosing instead to focus on the various treatments. They stood silently now, hands clasped, heads down. After a few moments of silence, Steven's daughter spoke. "My dad wouldn't want to live on machines," she said. "But if he could get back to his life, I know he'd want us to do everything."

None of her father's many problems were lethal in and of themselves. His body and brain simply hadn't improved. I couldn't tell her with confidence what would happen, but someone this sick for this long usually doesn't get better. But my own ICU reflexes were aroused, and truth be told, I didn't feel that I was ready to concede that death was a certainty. He had youth on his side and no obvious condemning diagnosis. And I had just met him. So I proposed, for all of our comfort, that we consider doing a time trial.

A *time trial*, or time-limited therapy, is a concept that has been discussed intermittently in the ICU and palliative care literature for a few decades. It is a period of time agreed on by the medical team and the family, by the end of which more clarity about prognosis is expected. A meeting is scheduled with the intention of regrouping, rethinking, reassessing. This date also sets a clear point at which families may consider changing goals of care.

Initiating a time trial alerts the family to the uncertainty rife in medicine. It sends the important message that we do not definitively know how things will evolve, even if we intend to come out of the gate with the full-court press. It prepares the family for the fact that we believe their loved one might die.

Time trials can also help physicians, who may not yet be ready to declare a prognosis but wish to communicate concern about the future. That can be helpful for both professional and emotional reasons, as I experienced in this case.

I see time trials as an opportunity for everyone to move from the minutiae of data, labs, and medication dosages to a 30,000-foot view of the situation. These trials offer an opportunity to take stock and see things from a different perspective. Two points on a graph—where we were and where we're going—can sometimes tell a very illuminating story. But this technique is too rarely used in the ICU. Dr. Doug White, an ICU researcher, found that out of seventy-two family conferences for patients at high risk of death in the ICU, time trials were offered only 15 percent of the time, and even in those cases, they were infrequently and incompletely discussed.

Standing outside Steven's room, I recommended to his daughter and son-in-law that we wait several days to see whether he might improve. If he continued to worsen, he would almost certainly eventually die. In that case, the daughter said, she was confident that the breathing tube should be removed. Her father would not want to live a compromised life—even the possibility of life on dialysis wasn't something she was sure he would accept.

If he stayed the same or improved, both unlikely scenarios, we would rethink next steps, consider a trach, and determine an interval for the next time trial.

There is no clear scientific method to selecting the time interval; it depends on the patient's condition, functional status, co-existing illnesses, and rate of decline. Ideally, it will take place at least several days before the two-week trach point, that weighty decision point. Sometimes, depending on the clinical certainty and the values of the patient and family, the time trial might end sooner; in other cases, it is appropriate to continue the time trial past the trach insertion.

When we regrouped a few days later, Mr. Cook was indeed worse. The family knew that even before we met because they had been watching the proceedings through a new lens and thus were asking different questions of the team and the nurses. The rest of the family had been alerted and was at the hospital on the day that we removed his breathing tube. Steven went on to live another forty-eight hours with high-level palliative and nursing care. He did not wake up, but he died peacefully with his family around him.

Time trials bring people together to help them do the right thing for the patient. Because of their very existence, a team has been formed, where all the players—the health care team, the family, the patient if he is able—are working toward a common goal: making a decision in real time that will avert as much suffering as possible for the patient. There is room for hope but the possibility of death has also been acknowledged; this lends time for the processing of emotions and information and eases future communication. The doctor has committed to reconnecting with the family with more information in order to reflect together on next steps.

Nobody is abandoned—neither the patient nor his loved ones.

Do What's Right for the Patient

Alma Lopez was blown up like an overfilled balloon. Ovarian cancer is known to cause terrible bowel obstructions, and this case was particularly bad. She hadn't had a bowel movement for at least two weeks. Granted, she wasn't eating much, but even saliva needs to pass through. The CT scan showed a severely distended small intestine due to a high-grade obstruction farther along its length. Food, liquid, and air were trapped and backing up.

As the palliative care consultant I was asked to help manage the patient's severe nausea and vomiting. She had been in and out of the hospital the previous week for the same problem, at which point she had been told that there were no further treatments to shrink the tumor. She had decided to return to her native Guatemala to die and had booked a flight for the next week. But now it wasn't clear she'd be well enough to go.

By the time I met her, she had stopped vomiting. The medical team had placed a nasogastric tube, which passed in through one nostril down to her stomach. The end of the tube was attached to a canister on the wall, which generated gentle suction to relieve some of the pressure. Almost a liter of stomach contents sat in the canister, and she told me she felt much better now. But I knew this was just a temporary solution. Almost as soon as the nasogastric tube was removed, she would be in the same place again. And despite her small improvements, her intestines were still filled with large amounts of fluid that could not fully be removed by the small tube.

In some cases of intestinal obstruction, doctors might consider a venting gastrostomy tube, which is placed directly through the skin into the stomach to allow air and fluid to escape. It usually remains in place permanently and is more effective at removing stomach contents than the temporary nasogastric tube. Yet it hadn't been considered as an option for Alma, who had already declared that her goals of care were to be kept comfortable. We often hesitate to perform procedures on fragile patients who have chosen to take a palliative approach. But there were two reasons why it made sense for Alma. First, she would have the ability to open the gastrostomy tube and drain her stomach whenever the pressure became uncomfortable. More comfort and more control; that seemed to be aligned with her goals of care. Second, Alma wanted to go home to die. I worried that if she did get on the plane to Guatemala, her bowel could rupture in the low pressure atmosphere of the cabin. And so, even though the surgery had risks, I suggested to the team that we offer the venting tube to her.

The team was uncomfortable. "But she's comfort care only," the resident stated, looking quizzical. "She has already said that she doesn't want to be treated aggressively or have her life prolonged artificially."

I provided my vision of stomach deflation. "The patient is so uncomfortable. She has temporary improvements when we put a tube through her nose into her stomach, but she goes right back to where she was as soon as it's taken out. If we put this vent in, her quality of life will be significantly improved." I also pointed out the disturbing image of an internal explosion of her bowels on an airplane. Still skeptical, the resident nodded when I suggested speaking with the interventional radiologists.

I went downstairs to Radiology. "We can definitely try, but isn't she comfort care?" the interventionist asked. He was known for his willingness to perform risky procedures if he thought they would benefit the patient. He took pride in his craft and was usually successful in his efforts. His hesitation here was out of character but not surprising. He saw himself as a saver of lives, an aggressive healer who could dive in and fix a problem urgently. But when it was in the context of impending death, he was uncomfortable. His work was about keeping people alive, not helping them die more comfortably. I wondered if it almost felt like a waste to him. All that work, only to be buried with the patient in the next several weeks.

When I explained the patient's goal of making it home to Guatemala, and the risks of air travel, he agreed to do it. Decompression was needed, and it would be good patient care. But we both knew it could make her worse. Alma was so fragile she might even die. We went upstairs together and presented the pros and cons of the procedure to her—continue this way with recurrent admissions and no trip home, or take a risk that could significantly improve her symptoms, but might mean dying. She weighed her options and decided to have the surgery.

I came to see Alma the next day, right after her procedure. The physician's assistant on our team was standing outside the room, looking concerned. "The nurse is in there with her. She's not doing well. She's vomiting a lot and I'm wondering if this was too aggressive. She just wanted to be comfortable." I noticed a touch of frustration in her voice. She had not been in support of the procedure and thought the risks outweighed the benefit. Then I learned that the gastrostomy tube's placement had triggered severe, nonstop vomiting. "I'm worried she will aspirate," said my colleague. Alma had put out almost four liters of gastric contents mixed with stool, she told me. It sounded dreadful and I felt a surge of concern that my approach had been wrong. I had wanted to help her live more comfortably and get to Guatemala, but had I instead accelerated her looming death?

Her room, though spattered with body fluids, was surprisingly quiet. Alma was sitting upright in a chair as her nurse busily changed the sheets on her bed. "There was an explosion here," said her nurse with a smile. "But we've got it under control." With the stomach contents ejected, the pressure was normalized and Alma was able to experience a level of comfort long forgotten. She gave me an exhausted smile and the biggest gift ever: a thumbs-up.

She was able to keep her reservation and fly home to Guatemala the following week. She died peacefully a few months later, among family, her pain and discomfort well managed during her final days.

We didn't know what would happen when we performed the venting gastrostomy. It could have gone either way. Had Alma suffered more, or died, I suspect I would have questioned my judgment as a palliative care practitioner. Happily, she did well, and so I allowed myself to feel good about my actions. But in truth, I would like to feel that I did the right thing by offering Alma the venting gastrostomy tube regardless of the outcome. It was her choice, after all, made with a fair representation of the various outcomes. It was shared decision making, something I always want to be proud of, regardless of the outcome.

Bernie Lown—Challenging Tradition

Residents who trained in internal medicine at the Brigham and Women's Hospital in the early 1990s remember the two different groups of cardiologists who walked the halls. One group consisted of the Brigham-based cardiologists, who cared for most of the inpatients on the wards. The other was the Lown Group, a private, mostly outpatient cardiology practice that admitted its patients to the Brigham as needed. Lown cardiologists had been trained under Bernard Lown, who had trained at the Brigham himself years before. Lown was responsible for developing the DC defibrillator in collaboration with Baruch Berkowitz, an electrical engineer. Their goal had been to find a current safer than AC to shock the heart back into rhythm during sudden cardiac arrest. And thus was born the modern symbol of life saving. "All clear! Shock at two hundred joules!" is a refrain now heard all around this country, in hospitals, ambulances, and on TV screens. The Lown Cardiovascular Group first used the defibrillator in the early 1960s on patients in the very same wards I would walk thirty years later.

Yet despite his contribution to the high-technology culture birthed in the mid-twentieth century, Dr. Lown's main focus was on the patient, not on the treatment. Lown refused to cleave blindly to the love affair that was taking place at that time between modern medicine and technology. Although his invention of the DC defibrillator—a staple in every hospital and ICU—earned him accolades, he was not willing to join in the unfettered celebration of technology. Dr. Lown went on to establish a cardiology practice that was very different from the status quo. And as a resident at the Brigham, it was impossible to ignore the difference.

While the regular attendings and cardiology fellows were teaching us to use Swan-Ganz catheters and other very invasive, technologically sophisticated interventions, the Lown cardiology fellows and attendings were trying to help us understand how to, in the words of Bernie Lown, "Do as much as possible FOR the patient and as little as possible TO the patient." In the occasional event that a Lown patient was deemed to need an invasive procedure, she was sent to the regular—at the time I thought of it as the *real*—cardiology service.

I look back on those days and remember my own inner dialogue about these two different types of doctors. The Lownies were nice guys, happy to sit down and teach a resident. I assumed they had more time to talk because they were doing less. The other cardiology group's fellows and attendings tended to be more brusque, not as attentive or patient, but always on hand to perform a procedure. It was a relief to have them show up at the bedside of a crashing patient—they were probably going to "do something." My original dismissal of the Lownies as inferior, softer, and less heroic stings me now. Without a doubt, today I would choose this group to provide my medical care. In fact, at my referral, both my mother-in-law and sister-in-law are patients in that practice.

Recently, I spoke with Vikas Saini, the president of the Lown Institute and himself a Lown fellow a few years before my time at the Brigham. "There was a sense of disdain one sometimes encountered if our interpretation of the data was that a particular patient would not benefit from an intervention," he told me. "We were looked on as Luddites, maybe even weak."

I remember feeling that way exactly.

Dr. Saini said he felt the tide is now beginning to turn. "We don't feel actively shunned anymore," he told me.

Well, that's progress, right?

Where mainstream cardiology splintered its focus into increasingly discrete and disconnected technological tributaries, Dr. Lown aimed to always remember the patient, with a holistic attitude and a less invasive approach. He has actually criticized the overuse of the very technology that he created, the DC defibrillator.

To me, Bernard Lown is a real hero. Not only is he responsible for saving countless lives with his defibrillator, but his courage in focusing on humanistic principles above all else, despite pressures and opposition in medical culture, is truly inspiring. He never lost sight of what really matters—the patient.

I've watched many people die. Patients, family, friends. And, as you can glean from this book, far too many of them have been bad deaths. What makes a death bad? I think it depends on the person. A former colleague at Vital Decisions told me that her father, a "crusty old Italian," once told her that if he couldn't wipe his own backside, he didn't want to live even one more day. My own worst fear is being alone in a room, unable to communicate, unable to connect with my loved ones. Each person has her own needs and preferences around death, and attending to them, down to the smallest of details, can enhance the life of a dying person.

I recently visited the Zen Hospice Project (ZHP), a six-bed home in the Hayes Valley neighborhood of San Francisco. Originally opened in 1990 in response to the AIDS crisis, the Hayes Valley Guest House was redesigned and reopened in 2010 as a licensed residential care facility for the chronically ill. It has a twenty-four-hour nursing staff, all of whom are trained in mindful, compassionate care. I referred several patients there during my year on the palliative care service at UCSF, but I had never visited until recently.

The Zen Hospice Project is housed in a beautifully painted Victorian on a tree-lined street. The front door is heavy and carved, with a leaded glass window. From the moment that I walked into the house, I was smitten. Warm Persian area rugs, comfortable furniture in clusters, lamps, and a wood-carved banister. There was a scent of banana bread, and we followed our noses into the kitchen, which was large and sunny, painted in warm yellows and greens. Fresh herbs were drying in a vase in the corner. A basket of citrus fruit sat on the counter.

The chef welcomed us with a big smile. She was in the process of assembling food for one of the residents. He was in the final stages of his illness and had little to no appetite. But she described what she had prepared for him with the enthusiasm of a chef preparing a gastronomic sensation for a crowd of foodies. The portions were miniature and she had set them on a small plate in three distinct samplings, like a tiny flight of pureed food. Each portion was a unique and vibrant color, and they complemented one another in a gorgeous palette. A nurse entered the kitchen with a different patient's tray. It, too, held only a small plate. I noticed that this plate's three portions were completely uneaten except for tiny indentations from the tip of a fork. I asked the chef how it felt to cook food for people who could barely eat it. She smiled. It had been tasted, she said, that's what mattered. Her job was to make known that she was downstairs cooking for the patients, or "guests." That she cared. That she wanted them to experience whatever they could, and no more. No pressure to eat anything, and certainly not everything. Smelling, tasting a little, and feeling loved were all she hoped for from them.

Zen Hospice's six beds serve a very diverse population, averaging sixty people per year for an average stay of four weeks. While the cost of hospice care is covered by insurance or the government, food and lodging costs are not. Nonetheless, the Zen Hospice Project strives to be means-blind, relying on charitable contributions, support from the local university hospital and a charitable foundation, and whatever amount someone is able to pay. The level of care administered to each patient is independent of what he pays as well as his insurance status. Each one receives the same careful attention to his food preferences, his comfort, and his dignity.

I looked around, thinking of my patients in the ICU. The breathing tubes that sit in the center of a mouth, rendering it almost impossible to clean. The artificial nutrition that drips through plastic tubes that weave through their mouths and noses into their stomachs. The arms, threaded with IVs, clamped by blood pressure cuffs, and, finally, tied down to the bed rails to prevent the patient from ripping these foreign objects off their dying bodies. While there is certainly a role for ICU care in many instances, for those at the end of life, I wish for better.

The hospice philosophy is to help the dying die in as comfortable and warm an environment as possible. Zen Hospice kicks this concept up a notch, providing for its six residents an aesthetic experience at the end of life that contrasts dramatically with the anesthetic experience that is the dying process in modern medicine.

The next time I walked into the ICU, I couldn't help but notice how cold and fluorescent it felt.

Goals of Hair

My friend's mother was coming to the end of her grueling fight with breast cancer. I had helped arrange home hospice services for her in her final days. By then she had become so sick from the relentless chemotherapy that she was spending most of her time either vomiting or sleeping. But finally in hospice she was able to rest. The bed was pulled into the center of the living room and she held court with her family.

My friend pulled me aside a few days before her mother died. "My mother made me promise to make sure she never had any hairs growing on her chin. But now I'm seeing one growing. What should I do?"

When she had still been healthy, before the cancer, before all of this, the older woman had made her daughter promise to immediately pluck any hairs on her chin when she was on her deathbed. Even if she was in a coma. They laughed about it at various

EXTREME MEASURES

times over the years, the good, and then the bad, but she had meant it.

We ushered everyone from the room and shut the door. My friend shone a flashlight on her mother's chin to illuminate the culprit hair, then plucked it. Then she brushed her mother's hair and fastened it in a clip. She murmured into her mother's ear that she was on the job. The woman died a few days later, impeccably groomed, as she had wanted.

This request, made in an intimate exchange between mother and daughter, is an example of what my team and I refer to as "goals of hair." One might think that in these final days, a dying person wouldn't notice or even care about how she looked. That by the time she has become so weak she can no longer brush her hair, or comb down an unruly cowlick, it won't matter to her. But these little details, which may feel vain, or trivial, or a distraction from the real work of fighting disease, are a part of who we are. Losing the ability or strength to groom oneself can add a film of self-consciousness, sadness, or even despair to the suffering already present. And so I believe it is important to discuss with our loved ones these intimate, maybe embarrassing personal preferences. This conversation may someday enable someone to receive the gift of a bit of autonomy at a time when everything else may feel out of control.

We'll Talk About It Once and Then Never Again

My palliative care teammate and I were perched on opposite sides of Jada's bed, one of us at her feet, the other near her knee. It had taken a few days to get this woman to talk to us. When she first heard that we were from the palliative care service, she had shaken her head politely and asked us to leave. She did not want to talk about death or dying, she said. She wanted to live. We understood completely, we said. Most of what we do for patients is to help them to live better. Would it be okay if we came and checked on her tomorrow?

That had gone on for two days, and today she had finally allowed us in the room.

Jada was fifty-one, with metastatic breast cancer. It had appeared six years earlier and she had undergone a mastectomy, chemotherapy, and radiation to the region. But a year and a half ago, when her other breast developed a mass that began to break down the skin, she didn't want to go through it all again. She had a nineteen-year-old son and two jobs. And so she bandaged up her chest and went on with her life.

She finally came to the hospital when she could barely breathe. Her lungs were chock-full of cancer, and one of the masses compressed the right side of her heart so that it couldn't properly fill with blood. But she refused to talk to the team about whether she would want to be placed on a breathing machine if it came to that. Or receive CPR. Or consider hospice. She just wanted them to do what they needed to do, she said. When the team pressed her further, she became profoundly anxious and turned away. And so she was currently listed as a full code.

The team had called us to help with addressing goals of care as well as managing her profound shortness of breath. But because she wouldn't let us in the room at first, we had helped them manage her symptoms from the sidelines. She was now breathing more easily and had agreed to let us, "the symptom management people," get involved. It felt like a major step forward.

Perched on her bed, we celebrated the improvement in her symptoms. "What is most important for you now?" we asked. And she began to tell us about her son, her family, her church.

"Sounds like you really want to get back to all of that," my colleague said. Jada nodded. "Our goal is to do everything that we can to make that possible," she said. With that, Jada smiled.

Before we left her, my colleague put a toe into the advance care planning waters. She expressed her concern that if a breathing tube was inserted, it would be unlikely that Jada would ever breathe on her own again. How did Jada feel about the use of a breathing machine, she asked our patient. Panic rose in Jada's eyes. "I told you I don't want to talk about this," she whispered.

We left the room discouraged. Jada was not ready to envision, let alone discuss, her death. And although she was exhausted, sad, anxious, and angry, she was clinging desperately to her life. Yet we were convinced she didn't want to die on the machine, which was exactly where she was headed at this point. Her panicked response at the suggestion, her avoidance of hospitals, her strong desire to be with her family—all pointed to a woman who did not want this kind of death. Yet it seemed too much for her to say those words herself; it would mean admitting she was dying. In our powerful desire to honor her autonomy, we wanted to hear her wishes from her own lips. But we realized that we wouldn't. She just couldn't go there.

In reflecting on the case, we realized that Jada did not want to be the driver here. It seemed to us she needed her doctors to lay out her care plan based on the clues she had given us and to guide her through it without too much discussion. She was alert, able to communicate clearly, and understood everything we were saying, and thus I felt we were unlikely to override her preferences. And of course if she disagreed with our navigation plan, we would jump to honor her preferences. But someone needed to make a move here, and it seemed to be us.

The next morning, we came by again. To our relief, she was

holding steady on the face mask, although she looked tired. Her brother was sitting next to the bed. We waved from the door and asked if we could come and visit. She didn't answer, but she didn't turn us away either. Her brother waved us in. "She's feeling strong today," he said. The patient gave a slight nod.

We settled on either side of her bed. "I'm so glad you're breathing on your own," my colleague said. "You are an incredibly strong woman. It seems like our medications are keeping you comfortable."

Another nod.

"We will keep treating any symptoms that come up and make sure to keep you off the breathing machine, okay? I know that is something you really don't want."

The patient looked at her, blinked, and then nodded.

"We will do everything we possibly can to help make you feel better, and stay away from treatments that will make things worse. No shocks or CPR." She didn't respond, just turned her head away. Then she asked her brother to pass her the water pitcher.

And that was it. She was alert and oriented—all she would need to do if she disagreed was shake her head. We didn't insist that she elaborate, sign anything, or even say, "Okay." We just moved forward and told her about all of the treatments that we *were* going to be doing, treatments that would almost definitely help her feel better and allow her to be with her family. The low-dose morphine would keep her shortness of breath under control, the steroids would help minimize the inflammation from the tumors. We talked about hospice without mentioning the sometimes emotionally laden name—instead, we described the hospital bed and equipment that would be brought in for her comfort, the trained nurses, and the emotional support for her brother and son. We did not focus again on what we would *not* be doing. The

DNR order was then signed into the chart and we warned the medical team and the nurse not to bring up code status with her again. She had made her decision known to us.

I have thought a good deal about this case. We are so much more comfortable when we hear specific instructions from a patient's lips. Yet I believe that some things are just too hard for some people to say.

While shared decision making has become my new gold standard, I have come to realize that there is no one-size-fits-all approach. A traditional exchange, where the doctor presents information and options and the patient actively selects her choice, occasionally needs to be supplanted by a more delicate dance, where the doctor must listen carefully for what remains unsaid. Jada didn't want to talk about things that scared her. Instead, I am convinced, she wanted her needs intuited.

Jada went home to her brother's house with hospice. Her brother took family medical leave in order to care for her, her son stayed by her side, and she spent her last days with her family. That is exactly what I believe Jada wanted, even if she wasn't able to say it outright. And if we had required that she do so, we would have committed her to a death I don't believe she wanted.

Acknowledging the Hidden Curriculum

It was the first week of Jenny's internship, and she was on my service in the ICU. During introduction on the first day, she expressed her excitement. She loved the ICU, she said, the procedures and the hustle-bustle of acute care. In medical school, the ICU rotation had been her favorite and she was planning to become an anesthesiologist and ICU attending herself one day.

A few days into the rotation, Jenny had a run of patients who did not do well. Two deaths over three days. During rounds on the fourth morning, I learned that another of her patients, a homeless man who had been dying for many days, had succumbed to his illness. As we were walking out of the conference room back toward the intensive care unit, I asked her how she was doing. She stood next to me, silent, looking straight ahead. This was unusual; she was generally cheerful, even peppy. I waited. Then she gasped and began to cry. She did her best to stifle it, wiping at her eyes and fanning her face. "I'm so sorry," she said, trying to laugh. "I'm not sure what got into me."

I ushered her to the side of the hallway. "It's completely okay," I said to her in a low voice. "You're allowed to feel things. It's what will make you a wonderful doctor. Please do not apologize."

She nodded briskly. "I didn't realize this was going to be so hard," she said to me. "I'm not sure I want to work in an ICU anymore."

I checked in with her a few times that week but she didn't seem to want to talk about it. Instead, she assumed her previous chipper demeanor.

Jenny wan't alone in her distress—or in her sense that it should be repressed. There is increasing awareness that the current medical education process has a hidden curriculum, discussed in the previous chapter, which comes into effect after the second year of medical school. During the formal curriculum of the first two, classroom-based years, the principles of humanism, patient-centeredness, and cultural sensitivity are processed in classroom cases, with supportive guidance and reflection. Attention is paid not only to the needs of patients, but to those of the learners, too. The clerkship years, however, occur in real time, with real patients, with the complex and nuanced circumstances you have read about in this book. There are no built-in mechanisms to provide support to trainees as they face real suffering—their patients' as well as their own.

The students' clerkship mentors are busy subspecialty physicians whose charge is to teach competence in the physiology and procedures of surgery, obstetrics, or other organ-focused fields. These doctors often do not have the time, or the proclivity or training, to reflect on the humanistic aspects of a given case. As a result, many medical students begin to emulate the behaviors of the only role models they see, usually doctors who themselves have been raised in this imperfect system and do not have a frame of reference for patient-centered care.

Research has demonstrated that the discordance between the formal and hidden curricula—specifically, when students witness supervisors practicing in ways contrary to those taught in school—has negative consequences for students' commitment to ethical principles as well as to their emotional well-being.

The December 2015 issue of the *Journal of the American Medical Association* focuses almost entirely on medical training, with an emphasis on the environmental pressures that form young physicians. The trauma of medical training is reflected in cartoons drawn by medical students at the Penn State College of Medicine; nearly half of them depict their attending physicians as abusive monsters. One drew a picture of a trainee urinating on herself in fear, with her head bitten off by her attending in the next panel. It should come as no surprise that medical trainees suffer staggering rates of depression: 28 percent compared with 16 percent in the general population.

The sense that emotions don't belong on the wards is another problem. In a recent study, 673 students from thirty-one medical schools across the nation were asked to identify aspects of themselves that they felt uncomfortable revealing in their training. The most common words used were *creativity, family, balance, freedom, peace, love, compassion, reflection,* and *relationships.* This was surprisingly stable across differing schools, years, and genders, suggesting that this problem is pervasive in medical training. The authors write:

> *If young doctors lose their sense of calling and creativity, medicine's capacity to respond to the health challenges of the future becomes severely limited. The pressure to suppress core personal values and qualities may help explain the frequently reported growth in cynicism, depression, and stunted moral growth observed as medical students progress through their training.*

Medical culture accepts this transformation of the medical student as inevitable. Seasoned doctors, and even residents further along in their training, generally treat the incoming medical students with the attitude of a tough parent mentoring a child through the teenage years. There is an understanding that the child is suffering, but he will get through it. It is considered a normal part of the training process, even a rite of passage, to experience emotional distress, even to cry as Jenny did, but the expectation is that students must acclimate to this environment in order to continue on. And, goes the thinking, if we went through it, why should they be spared? There is a punitive element to this but also the sense that in order to make it in this profession, the kids need to toughen up. It is a culture of trauma, and it is passed from generation to generation.

But an awareness of these deficits in medical training has begun to percolate, beginning in the ivory towers of select medical schools. Programs such as The Healer's Art, which started at the University of California, San Francisco in 1991 and has been adopted by eighty U.S. medical schools to date, aim to support humanism in medical training. The Healer's Art is an opt-in program that encourages mindful reflection, deep listening, and storytelling, aiming to enable students to uncover and strengthen the altruistic values that led them to medicine in the first place. This program acknowledges the intrinsic difficulty of caring for the gravely ill, allowing students to sit with that difficulty instead of leaping to fix it.

I believe programs like these should not be an opt-in offering, but rather a required element of the medical curriculum. These concepts should be taught not only as part of the formal curriculum but provided throughout the clerkship years, when students are even more in need of support, reflection, and patient-centered role models. This will require a significant restructuring of the existing medical education system. For now, let us begin with a separate, required clerkship that exists, equally valued, alongside the traditional rotations of medicine, surgery, and OB-GYN. This clerkship would rotate students through a broad variety of locations and specialties—the ICU, the oncology suite, and the geriatrics clinic—in order to demonstrate how to practice patient-centered medicine regardless of the specific medical problem or location. Faculty mentors from various subspecialty backgrounds would be trained to guide the students through this perilous terrain and bring this teaching philosophy back to their own clerkships.

Recently, I was talking to three local medical students about this idea. I started to tell them stories about difficult cases, ethically nuanced cases, in which I'd done the best I could and yet things still went badly. They stared at me dumbstruck. I began to feel worried that I had upset them, been too negative. But they shook their heads and thanked me. They didn't feel they had been prepared for what they would soon encounter on the wards. One mentioned she had noticed that almost all of the case discussions in her first year had happy endings. Patients either recovered or, if they died, there was no ethical conflict. They began to under-stand that their reflective and humanistic lecture halls had not prepared them for the shock of being on the medical wards the following year.

But here's the good news. Just as medical students and resi-dents can be changed by the hidden curriculum that exists on the wards, so too can they be a force for change. Each year brings a new crop of students and residents to our medical wards. An "in-oculation" such as The Healer's Art into traditional curricula might bring about significant change within a couple of years. When I think about the options available to the medical students who sat sipping tea in my dining room last month compared to when I was a student, I feel a surge of optimism about the future.

The shift toward more holistic training is under way. One example is VitalTalk, a nonprofit that teaches medical practi-tioners advanced communication skills, with the goal of enabling them to foster more robust connections with their patients. I completed their faculty training course recently and walked out feeling very hopeful. If their content became integrated into mainstream medical culture, I thought, it could change every-thing. Even the most basic of the skills they imparted were things we were never taught in medical school and certainly not on the hospital wards. Other initiatives are slowly emerging, like the Lown Institute's RightCare rounds, currently in its pilot phase. These rounds take the form of time-honored grand rounds but incorporate the patient's psychological and social history as well as what is known about her preferences and goals of care. The aim is to offer a more comprehensive context for these discus-sions, enabling patients to actively choose treatment approaches aligned with their values. Another example is Schwartz Center Rounds, initiated in 1995 to encourage compassionate care by supporting health care providers to have regular dialogues about difficult and emotional cases. They are now being practiced in 375 health care institutions in the United States.

Times are indeed changing. Hang in there, Jenny.

PADDLES

In 2007, Atul Gawande's essay "The Checklist" appeared in *The New Yorker*. In it, Dr. Gawande makes the convincing argument for using checklists in medicine, where the complex and high-stakes environment is rife with the potential for error.

After reading it, I began to wonder how many things I might be missing in the care of my patients. Despite careful rounding, we occasionally delayed or even, although rarely, failed to offer interventions that might save lives—for example, medication to prevent stomach ulcers or blood thinners to protect against blood clots. These preventive measures might seem mundane, but they can be crucial. We were doing a great job of putting in lines, diagnosing illnesses, and managing breathing machines, but we sometimes missed the easier, more obvious treatments.

Instead of putting the blame on my overwhelmed interns and residents, on the pharmacy, or on myself, I created a checklist that, after multiple iterations with input from many resident teams, I named PADDLES. Although far from perfect, it incorporated most of what I thought we needed. After residents presented each patient's list of medical problems, I would ask, "And what about PADDLES?" They would stumble through the list, haltingly, until they'd memorized it. But by the end of the rotation, if the case was uncomplicated, they could complete it within forty-five seconds.

P stands for prophylaxis and includes the blood thinners and stomach protectant I mentioned earlier. *A* stands for alimentary, or nourishment. Should the patient be receiving tube feeds or fluids at this time? The first *D* stands for delirium, a highly prevalent, frequently missed, and often treatable condition in ICUs that contributes greatly to suffering and mortality. The second *D* stands for disposition, meant to address some very important questions: Where do we go from here? What is the patient's prognosis? Who is making decisions, and what information needs to be shared? This is the most misunderstood part of the checklist, but it is critically important. I will come back to it in a moment.

L stands for lines: all of the lines that have been placed into the patient in order for us to access the bloodstream, bladder, lungs, and other hard-to-get-to places. It's important to keep track of these potential sources of infections and blood clots. *E* is for excruciating (this was a stretch, but bear with me). It is critical to treat pain in a person who is intermittently conscious and tied down in a bed on a breathing machine. And finally *S* stands for sedation, that crucial means of easing the anxiety and trauma of an ICU stay. Differentiating between pain and anxiety is essential in the care of an ICU patient. Pain receptors are different from those for anxiety, but if a doctor thinks that just because the patient is now quiet she has adequately managed the pain, she may be tragically mistaken.

That second *D* for disposition is the concept with which my teams tend to have the most difficulty. These are the thorniest issues of ICU care—the hard conversations, the breaking of bad news. The residents initially prefer to go concrete on me here, discussing the literal disposition plan. "The patient should obviously stay in the ICU, because she's still requiring the breathing machine," is a common response. But with redirection, they begin to understand that I am referring to a more fundamental, even existential meaning of the word. I find that as the week goes on, my residents become more comfortable with and willing to discuss these difficult topics.

It can feel awkward, at first, to focus on something as mundane as prophylaxis, when minutes before we'd been discussing our strategies for managing the patient's heart failure or hemorrhage. I worried my residents might feel insulted by my requiring them to check their work. And it took extra time—even an extra one or two minutes per patient can feel substantial to an overworked group of young residents. Yet I was surprised and delighted last year to see that PADDLES was written, with a description for each letter, at the top of the resident sign-out sheet in the ICU. It was being passed from resident to intern, and from outgoing to incoming. My residents had accepted this checklist and seen the value to their patients.

To me, this experience speaks volumes about the possibility for positive change in the ICU. It is refreshing to see residents embracing a process that is not flashy but, rather, mundane. And their humility in acknowledging that they are human and prone to forgetting will, I trust, benefit their patients.

An Experiential Tour Guide

In their third trimester, pregnant women usually go on tours of the labor and delivery suite. These tours serve many purposes—some logistical, some emotional, some simply cognitive. It is helpful to know where to park your car and what to pack in your suitcase. It is less scary to enter a hospital when you are physically compromised if you have been prepared for what will take place. And if you have plenty of advance time to consider what treatments will be right for you before pain, panic, or disorientation can take over.

Why don't we take chronically ill patients on tours of the ICU? I believe that if Uncle Barry or Vincent had seen what PEGs, trachs, and breathing machines look like when attached to patients who are dying, they might not have chosen to pursue the courses they did. But either way, I would have felt much better knowing that they had some visual sense of that state before they found themselves in it.

Advance Care Planning Decisions is a Boston-based company that produces videos which attempt to bring to life many of the treatments used in managing patients with serious illness. There are videos about CPR, chemotherapy, and ICU treatment, all in a multitude of languages. Co-founder Dr. Angelo Volandes recounts how, many years ago, he was the hospital attending for a woman with terminal cancer. Already possessing a particular interest in advance care planning, he tried to describe several of the procedures that might await her down the line. He had the feeling she didn't really understand what he was describing. And so he took her on a field trip. He asked her to walk down the hall with him to the ICU. Touring the space, she looked at him and shook her head. "Words, words, words," she said, and told him that while she had understood what he had said, she had to see it with her own eyes to get clear that she didn't want that type of treatment for herself.

The Marine

Don, a thirty-one-year-old salesman, had been suffering from cancer for eight years. Although he didn't yet realize it, he had entered the active phase of dying when I met him, returning to the hospital for the second time in two weeks. I was his palliative care physician, brought in to help manage his pain and symptoms.

The previous week, Don's thorax had been hastily punctured with chest tubes to remove some of the accumulated cancerous liquid around his lungs. Two days before I met him, the tubes had been removed, but the fluids had reaccumulated surprisingly fast. Don, a former Marine who served two tours of duty in Iraq, was now gasping for air. He was also suffering from severe nausea and constipation and was holding a basin up to his mouth to catch the vomit from his constant retching. A tall and broad-shouldered man, he had lost all his bulk; the angel he'd had tattooed on his shoulder to mark his fifth anniversary free of cancer had shriveled. His belly was distended, his face was gray, and his head was bald. His wife was beside him, gently wiping the spittle off his face.

Don's parents had flown to his bedside three days earlier. Together with his wife, they were supporting him through what they believed would be a six-month battle to keep him alive long enough to enroll in an experimental trial testing a new melanoma drug.

His doctors privately had their doubts that he could survive the six months, but had supported the patient's decision to "fight till I'm in the grave," as he had said months earlier. He was newly married with a lovely wife, and willing to do anything that might help his chances for survival. Treatment after invasive treatment had been tried over the previous several months of his rapid decline, but to no avail. In addition to Don's extreme shortness of breath, he suffered excruciating chest pain from inflammation at the site of the prior chest tubes. The nephrologist had also been called to evaluate the cause of his new kidney failure. After a few minutes of introduction, Don's father, a tall and authoritative military professional, pulled me into the hall and asked, "Where are we at this point?"

The question was vague. He might have been wondering what the next treatment would be. But his sad eyes told me the truth. He was starting to doubt that the cancer could be beaten. Until now, he had been supporting his son as he went through the battle, assuming the injuries and casualties were necessary collateral damage. But now I could tell he was starting to question whether there was a benefit to the suffering.

I responded with a series of questions. I didn't have all of the answers he needed, but I helped him pull together information about his son's medical status, available treatments, and, most important, about Don himself. I discussed the risks and benefits of the various options and helped him determine what information he needed from the oncologist. We talked about Don—his hopes, his plans, his wife. He told me that Don was proud, strong, and a real fighter. But, he said, Don also knew when to retreat. "He wouldn't stay in a battle if he was losing his men," he told me quietly.

As I huddled in the hallway with Don's father, the nephrologist emerged from the room. He acknowledged that Don's kidney failure was bad, and probably permanent, but reassured the father that dialysis could wait. But Don's father, now with a new need for clarity, asked directly whether kidney failure would exclude Don from the trial that was being planned. The nephrologist admitted that clinical trials rarely, if ever, accepted patients with kidney failure. He also added that he couldn't imagine that Don had more than a short period of time to live.

This was the moment of clarity Don's father needed. He drew a deep breath, wiped a tear from his eye, and thanked us for our honesty. The battle was lost, he said, and the time had come to concentrate instead on Don's comfort and dignity.

But when we talked to Don's wife, she vehemently disagreed. The oncologist would be back to check on Don's progress in two days, she said, and she didn't want to change the plan until she had heard from his lips that there were no other options. But I wasn't sure Don had two more days, I told her. He was failing rapidly. If the current course was to be maintained, within a day or two he would probably need a ventilator and medication to support his blood pressure. This decision would guarantee that he died hooked up to machines in an ICU. She was quiet. I suggested we call the oncologist in his clinic together, and she agreed. I dialed the number on the telephone speaker.

After ten long minutes on hold, the oncologist picked up. He was in a busy clinic, he said, and didn't have much time to talk. How could he help?

I explained that the family needed some clarity on Don's condition immediately, in order to make sure that the current plan was still appropriate. "Is there anything else to try," I asked him, "anything that will make a significant difference in his clinical course?" The oncologist hesitated. I imagine it was hard for him to acknowledge that there were no further life-prolonging treatments to offer this young man. He slowly began to list a few possible regimens, but then his voice trailed off. Don's wife and father, listening in to the conversation, looked hopeful. "Are any of those treatments used in patients with kidney failure?" I asked. The oncologist admitted that there were no further treatments for the cancer.

This was the moment of truth for Don's wife. She began to sob and said she didn't want him to suffer any longer. We began treating his symptoms more aggressively, and by the next day, his pain and vomiting had subsided enough for us to have a conversation. He received the news about his condition with grace. He wanted to go home, he told us, with what sounded to me like relief.

Unfortunately, he never left the hospital. After an unexpected complication, he died at 3:30 the next morning, in the comfort care suite of our hospital. But he was free from pain, at peace, and surrounded by his family. His wife was able to lie next to him for most of the night, her arms around him, feeling for each breath, whispering words of love and support. His mother, at first hysterical with grief, grew calmer knowing that his pain and suffering were under control. And his father sat stoically in a chair next to his son's bed, watching him with grief and pride.

In our eyes, Don was a hero to the end.

My Own Death

To me, in this profession, at its simplest level, heroism is acceptance of our own mortality. And that is where we all—doctors and laypeople alike—must draw on our courage.

I attended a conference called "Mindfulness in the ICU" at the University of California, San Francisco, several years ago. I was at once intrigued and baffled. At the time, the title of the conference struck me as an oxymoron. Can one be mindful in an ICU, where every second counts? Should one? Taking even a moment to breathe or to reflect seemed a bit risky to me at that time.

Yet I had been hearing more about mindfulness, a modern spin on meditation, and had even taken an eight-week course from StressCare, one of a number of new groups introducing this tool to the lay public. StressCare had been recruited to train residents and staff at UCSF, and so it felt like a legitimate, serious organization. Moreover, the conference was being led by Dr. Mitchell Levy, an ICU hero doctor if there ever was one. An associate professor of medicine at Brown University, Dr. Levy had been one of the lead investigators for the Surviving Sepsis Campaign in 2002, from which had emerged the widely accepted approach to managing critically ill patients with sepsis, one of the ICU's most common and lethal conditions. If he was the sponsor of this conference, it couldn't be too "out there" for me to try.

Dr. Levy was also the chair of the Robert Wood Johnson Foundation's critical care end-of-life workgroup. He had started lecturing about the lack of mindfulness among physicians, which he believed contributed to their problems in caring for their patients and for themselves. He believed that teaching mindfulness to clinicians would enhance their abilities to serve their patients by being able to hold space, slow down, and really listen. And he also postulated that if physicians learned to soothe themselves in their work environments—especially places like the fast-paced ICU—everyone, patient and physician, would do better.

In reading about him, I learned that Dr. Levy had been a practicing Buddhist since his college days. His bio stated that he was a senior teacher in the Shambhala Buddhist tradition and that he drew from his Buddhism in an effort to teach communication and compassion skills to medical professionals.

It was a daylong workshop and I arrived at 8:00 A.M. After the attendees grabbed coffee and Danishes, we were asked to take a seat in the main room. It was set up very differently from most conferences, the chairs in a large circle. Dr. Levy introduced himself and then asked people to go around the room introducing themselves to the group. I was disappointed, although unsurprised, to find that physicians were in a significant minority. Most of the people attending were nurses, with a smattering of physical therapists, respiratory therapists, and administrators.

Dr. Levy didn't look like a Buddhist, I thought. He looked like a doctor, with a blue suit and tie and white cropped hair. The only thing that struck me as Buddhist was that he had removed his shoes. Unusual, but it seemed quaint and lent an atmosphere of authenticity to the experience. He smiled at the group, slowly looking around the circle, acknowledging each of us individually. "Who here has pictured his or her own death?" he asked quietly. There was silence, then a few nervous chuckles. Then a couple of hands rose tentatively. Not mine. He went on. "How can we expect to help our patients plan for their deaths if we haven't planned for ours?" He waited, not so much for a response but for his words to sink in. The room was quiet, but Dr. Levy seemed to expect it. "I'd like us to do an exercise where we picture our own deaths," he said. "Who would be there? What would they be saying? Who would be crying? What would you have not gotten done? For what would you be grateful? Who would be holding your hand? Who would be standing at the foot of the bed? In the hall?" And with those instructions, he fell silent and closed his eyes. And so did we.

I realized that although I was around death every day, I had never before allowed myself to consider my own. It was as if I had willed myself immune to it.

But now I let it seep in. The sadness. The uncompleted tasks. The things I would miss. The weddings. The grandchildren I might never meet or see graduate. I saw my children crying. I saw their kids growing up without knowing me. I imagined my husband remarried, a new wife living in my house, stepmother to my children, grandmother to my grandchildren.

But then I began to consider whom I would want to be next to me. And what I would say to them. The words of encouragement, the instructions I would give them. I imagined the unknown, which may not be all bad. And the tears started to fall down my cheeks. One big fat one at first, brimming over and paving a salty track down my dry cheek to come to an embarrassing stop at the corner of my mouth. I wasn't sure if I should lick it or ignore it. And thus my mindfulness exercise ended because I needed all of my focus to suppress my impending sobbing. I was relieved when Dr. Levy took in a deep breath and rang a bell concluding the meditation. I had been saved from the mortification of being an ICU physician sobbing uncontrollably as I pondered my own death. And right in front of the nurses, physical therapists, and respiratory therapists that I feel I must stand before confidently, never wavering in my resolve that I can make it right for my patient.

In all my years of practice, it was the first time I had truly faced my own death. It's not that there hadn't been opportunity. Every year at the Rosh Hashanah (the Jewish New Year) service, I read aloud the prayer Unetaneh Tokef (Let Us Cede Power). This prayer attests to our lack of control over our mortality, willing us to repent and mend our ways in order to be inscribed in the Book of Life for another year. Its words are sobering, even grisly.

> *On Rosh Hashanah it is inscribed, and on Yom Kippur it is sealed:*
> *how many shall pass on, and how many shall be born;*
> *who shall live, and who shall die;*
> *who in his time, and who before his time;*
> *who by fire and who by water;*
> *who by sword and who by beast;*
> *who by hunger and who by thirst;*
> *who by storm and who by plague;*
> *who by choking and who by stoning . . .*
> *who shall rest, and who shall wander;*
> *who shall be tranquil and who shall be harassed;*
> *who shall be at peace and who shall suffer;*
> *who shall become poor, and who shall become rich;*
> *who shall fall and who shall rise . . .*

But somehow it never felt real. These types of deaths—by stoning, drowning, thirst, or sword—always felt strange, ancient, more of an attestation to ritual than to reality. They had nothing to do with me.

But sitting in that circle, I finally let it in, the hard fact of my mortality. Opening to the sadness, I realized I'd been running away from it. I began to think more deeply about how I would help all of those walking that path before me. How could I possibly help my patients accept their deaths if I hadn't stopped to accept mine?

I am, of course, no different from my patients, no better or worse. Often no wiser. And no more entitled to live another day. I reminded myself that death comes for us all, and sooner or later, I will be the one in that bed, on the other end of the stethoscope.

I considered what type of doctor I would want to have with me as I made these final decisions, as I breathed my final breaths. It would be one who would strive to know who I was and what was most important to me. One who would counsel my family members if I could not speak for myself. Who would alleviate my suffering, make sure I never felt abandoned or scared, that all of the pieces were in place. And then allow me to pass peacefully into that good night.

I opened my eyes and took a deep breath. I had my work cut out for me.

Epilogue

Marcia Green

Marcia Green had sprung a leak. And now she was having trouble breathing. The CT scan showed a left lung that was compressed into a tight ball by a large amount of fluid in her chest cavity. The liquid had likely accumulated over time, as she had been having symptoms for at least ten days. Sinister-looking mounds of tissue had infiltrated other organs. This was definitely not good.

Marcia had been diagnosed with lung cancer the previous year, but she now told the doctors, with some relief, that it had been taken out, cured. And because doctors are trained to keep quiet until they have all of the facts, she had no idea that her death was unfolding in front of her eyes.

Although it had not yet been confirmed under the microscope, her case was not mysterious to us. Four months of unintended weight loss, weakness, and blood-tinged sputum. A suspicious lung mass in a person with a history of lung cancer. A new pleural effusion. This was right out of Harrison's textbook of medicine. While indeed the initiating lung cancer had been surgically removed the previous year, some of the cancer cells had remained, steadily spreading through her body. Most doctors have taken care of patients like Marcia. By the time they get to us, it is a rapid downward descent. Chemotherapy almost never helps. If anything, it saps whatever life is left in the body.

The doctors drained the fluid, both to ease her breathing and to send a sample to the pathologists for confirmation of the diagnosis. As the wine-colored liquid sprayed into the collection bottle, Marcia transformed, a resident later told me. "I can take a deep breath again," she told the team. "Haven't been able to do this for weeks. You doctors are amazing!"

However, the next day she couldn't walk across the room. The fluid had reaccumulated shockingly quickly. Her doctors decided to place a PleurX tube, permanent and surgically perched between two ribs, which could be drained a few times a day to treat shortness of breath. She would be able to open the spigot to release the fluid and obtain relief again.

When the diagnosis was revealed, metastatic lung cancer with a malignant pleural effusion, she was told that she would receive chemotherapy to minimize the effusion. She went home with a plan. Report to the oncology clinic to receive her chemotherapy once a week for the next six weeks. And release fluid from the PleurX no more than twice a day, up to a half liter as necessary for worsening shortness of breath. Both instructions felt like something to do, and although she realized that neither was a cure, she was still in the fight. She left the hospital believing she had years left to live.

I first met her in the ICU on her next admission. She had been admitted in profound shock, with a dangerously low blood pressure. She hadn't understood that it was extremely dangerous to release more fluid than instructed, as she might unintentionally drain the vascular system of all of its pressure. The doctors had assumed that chemotherapy would work and diminish the accumulation of fluid. But they had been wrong. Since discharge, she had been removing an enormous amount of fluid from her pleural space, half a liter two to three times a day, about a quarter of her body water per week. Even more worrying, a lot of the fluid was blood, making her seriously anemic on top of being in shock. She was like an open spigot, constantly pouring, even when she was sleeping.

We got to work quickly, snaking a large catheter into a neck vein for rapid infusion of blood and fluids. She started to rehydrate, like one of those animal-shaped sponges in dissolvable capsules you give your kids in the bath. The corners of her mouth, which had hung on her face like two south-pointing arrows, now defied gravity again, sometimes achieving a tired smile.

She had barely stabilized before her children converted her room into command central. It was time to fight again, they said. I imagined them at ringside, a quick infusion of saline and anti-nausea medication, a dose of morphine for her aching chest, a slap on the back as she limped into the ring for another pummeling by poisonous medicine. But this fighter didn't look like she could even limp. In fact, she couldn't get out of bed. Just using the bedpan was a three-person affair, with a lot of wincing and shifting of tubes and gear. And because earlier chemotherapy had not worked as intended, I couldn't imagine another concoction would work any better, especially in her current debilitated state.

Marcia knew something was wrong. She didn't know how to say it to her children, but she couldn't keep going this way. Our

ICU toolbox had righted her ship, but she knew it was only a matter of time before the next capsize. She could feel the constant oozing of blood and fluid into her chest, she told me, feel it rising up around her left lung and compressing it. Her own body turning on itself. The chemotherapy she'd been taking for months was becoming unbearable. At first, she'd been able to push through the nausea, vomiting, and fatigue by picturing her grandbaby awaiting her return. But the last several infusions had been brutal, each familiar side effect increasingly dreaded. The idea of doing it again was simply too much.

But how could she tell this to her children? Her daughter, who depended on her for babysitting, cooking tips, counsel. Her son, whose wife was pregnant with their first child. Both so proud of their mom fighting to stay alive.

As the ICU attending, my job was to save her life. I had done that. No longer actively dying, she had earned the "no longer appropriate for the ICU" label. Our job was done. And we really needed the bed. The ER was jammed up and there were two patients on ventilators waiting to come in. Marcia's nurse had already given the report to the step-down unit and had accepted a report from the ER nurse for a different patient.

But in watching this drama, I realized that I hadn't done my job. And I knew from ample experience that if I didn't tell her she was dying now, she might never be told. And this woman had run out of time.

Gathering my residents and the harried nurse around me, I told them I was holding up the transfer. Blank stares. A tapping foot. "What is going to happen to Marcia after she leaves here?" I asked.

A resident volunteered the obvious. "She'll finish her last chemotherapy treatment. Then we'll see if it is helping."

I turned toward the well-meaning doctor. "She's had five of

the six courses of chemo, and her pleural effusion has gotten significantly worse. She's already had all of the radiation to the area that she can have. How likely is it that more chemotherapy will help?"

I felt the stirrings of a mutiny from my stressed residents. "Can't the medical team do this once she gets up to the wards? Give the family another day to get comfortable with what's going on?"

"Things could deteriorate very rapidly," I said. "We need to do it now, while she can still talk to us."

Her daughter, Amanda, nodded to us as we entered the room. Heavyset, with a direct gaze, this woman clearly did not suffer fools. She was facing this thing head on, uninterested in exchanging pleasantries. She was in the middle of giving her mother a "strengthening massage with pressure points for the nausea," she explained tersely. I thought of boxers being massaged by their managers before being pushed into the ring. Marcia gave me a tired smile. Everything about her was giving in to gravity. Her hair hung around her face, and her eyelids were heavy. She didn't look as if she could handle the news I was bringing. This poor woman was spent.

My residents shifted nervously and kept to the back of the room. The nurse watched from the other side of the glass door. This was not a typical conversation to be having with a patient who had improved enough to be transferred out, and everyone knew that it might throw a wrench into the day's work.

There was no chair, so I asked Marcia if I could perch on the end of her bed.

"Of course. Make yourself comfortable," she said. Her voice was quiet, barely audible.

The plastic mattress was slippery, even though covered with the hospital sheet, and emitted a puff of air as I sat on it. "We've gotten you stabilized for now," I said, and watched as they registered my last two words. "We don't need to keep you in the ICU at this point, and we have a bed waiting for you upstairs."

"That's good . . . ?" Her words had a questioning lilt. Amanda had stopped rubbing and looked ready to eject me from the room. *There's no space for negativity here,* her eyes said.

"I want to make sure that we're all on the same page about what's happening," I said. "What do you understand about your cancer?"

Marcia concentrated on a fold in her hospital gown, straightening it to lie parallel to its neighbor. I waited. Everyone waited. Finally, she looked at me and took a deep breath. "I know I'm sick, but I just need another five years. I'm not greedy. Just some time to settle my husband and kids."

We both knew she didn't have five years. She would be lucky, in fact, to have another few months, given the aggressive nature of her cancer and the physiologic instability of her fluid loss.

Twenty years I've been doing this now and it has never gotten any easier. It wasn't too late to send her off to the waiting bed with some rallying words. I could think of many reasons to do that, and many excuses to explain it to my residents and the nurses. I was tired and very busy, and we needed her bed.

But then I thought of those whom I had followed to this moment, this bedside—my father, my uncles, my immigrant grandparents who had worked themselves to the bone to get me to this bedside. I wanted to make them proud. Pat, Dr. Connors, Dr. Levy. Theirs were giant footsteps to walk in. But this small step, I knew, was taking me in the right direction. This was what I could give right now, meager as it felt.

I looked her in the eyes and spoke the truth as gently as I could. "Your cancer has reached a very serious stage," I said. "There are no more curative options for us to try. Chemotherapy hasn't worked, and at this point it will just make you sicker than you already are. There are no surgeries or other treatments that can keep the cancer at bay."

My patient's tight smile slackened, and she exhaled a slight "Oh." Amanda's hands, which encircled her mother's thin wrists, sat motionless on the pressure points.

I waited, letting the news sink in. When she realized her eleven-month-old granddaughter would not know her, she began to cry. I let her sadness pour over me, my own tears brimming over, and held her hand as she sobbed. I imagined the burden that this dying woman had been carrying, and I could only hope that the truth brought its own kind of relief.

As her crying ebbed, the room became silent. Amanda's hands had dropped to her sides, and her eyes were cast down. I began to gently probe for ways we could best support them now, but they remained quiet. And so I began to offer a vision for a different kind of hope. I talked of achieving the best life possible in the time that remained, the one most closely aligned with her own values and priorities. I brought up the concept of hospice, which would allow her to receive excellent symptom management in her own home. I was determined to show them that we would continue to support them, not just send them off to deal with this on their own. I began to describe the many things that we could do for her right now, the strategies to enhance the precious time she had left.

When I had finished, they nodded and thanked me. I walked out of the room wondering if I had made the wrong decision after all. Had my news devastated this family beyond recovery?

Twenty-four hours later, when I visited her room on the medical ward, the answer was clear. The funereal tone of yesterday had given way to palpable relief. The mood was almost celebratory. "Hey there, doc," Marcia said, grinning, as she opened her arms to receive a hug. Marcia and her husband were making a to-do list in consultation with Amanda, whose face bobbed on the iPad screen on Marcia's lap. And this list was refreshingly achievable. It included things like ordering a case of her favorite wines to sample with friends, organizing her photo albums, and purchasing board games. Notably absent were the tasks from yesterday's list: the toxic treatments, the plan for a vacation in Hawaii, the follow-up visits to various clinics.

Marcia sat in her wheelchair smiling from ear to ear. "We've decided to go for hospice. The team is already setting it up. Come look at this, Dr. Zitter," she said with excitement, pointing to the iPad on her lap. "Amanda has set up my bed in the living room so that if I get tired, I can still be with the family." Amanda, always businesslike, called to her impatiently. "Mom! Which one should I open?" She turned the camera to the table, where three bottles of wine stood in a row. "Let's do the cab, sweetie," Marcia said. "And make sure to decant it now so that we can have a nice glass when I get home."

This switch in direction may seem abrupt, and in a way it was. But it makes sense. This family had been running on fumes—of adrenaline and false hope. They were a highly organized and motivated bunch. They had summoned all of their resources to fight this battle, but I believe that on some level they had begun to suspect the truth. Stopping would have felt disloyal, as if they didn't love their mother enough. They needed permission from a doctor. Now that the abscess of secrecy had been drained, every-one was relieved to move forward.

Marcia knew what she wanted to do with the time she had left. Chemotherapy was off the table—100 percent and no look-ing back. If she'd made that decision twenty-four hours earlier, she told me, it would have signaled despair and hopelessness. But now she was excited to lift the chains of that treatment and move on to different options that focused on quality of life. We all agreed that prophylactic radiation treatment to her brain was a reasonable treatment to pursue. Less toxic and life disrupting than chemotherapy, it might help keep the metastases in the base of her brain small and prevent new ones from arising over the next several weeks to months of her life. If she didn't tolerate it, we'd stop. But the most powerful therapy for her was family time, and she knew that she didn't want to spend one more day in the hospital. Her main logistical goal was to sell her house and move to Pleasant Hill, where Amanda's family lived, so that her husband would not be alone after she died. She shifted up the dates for packing and moving so that she could get set up quickly, before she began to deteriorate again.

She got four good weeks at home. They got the house sold "by the grace of God," as she put it, and planned for her husband to move in with Amanda when the time came. She checked everything off her list before she died. And had a lot of fun too. She played Scrabble with her children, snuggled with her grandchildren in her hospital bed, and drank some good wine.

I went to the funeral. It was a beautiful tribute to a life well lived. The church was filled to the brim. The family seated me in a place of honor and thanked me repeatedly for giving them the time with her that they had. Every minute was a gift, her son said. There were many people who spoke of her love of life, her passion, and her will to live every minute of her life to the fullest. This funeral was a celebration of her life.

I see so many patients, so many lives. Very few have this opportunity to live life all the way through to the end. So many are cut off from life before their bodies leave this earth. We've achieved amazing things in modern medicine. Our tools can bring the dying back to life. But too often they serve to take life away from the dying. I sat at that funeral with tears streaming down my face. But these were not tears of failure or even grief.

They were tears of joy. This is what life should be, right to the end. This is what I want my funeral to look like—my loved ones celebrating my passion, my joie de vivre—in short, how I had *lived*.

Amanda spoke of Marcia's last day, which was filled with family. She died in my arms, she said, and it was as loving and peaceful a death as she could imagine. A gift I'll be forever grateful for, she said. *Yes,* I thought, wiping my eyes. *That's the kind of death I want for myself.*

On that afternoon, I felt like a hero.

A Way Forward

M ANY PEOPLE SEE advance care planning for the end of life as a one-stop shop. They file their Advance Directives away in the safe deposit box, alongside wills and homeowner's insurance, and believe they are done. Not so. In my experience, the best-laid paths to the end of life have been paved with ongoing reflection and communication.

Research demonstrates that as people approach death, whether from advancing age or disease, their priorities shift—sometimes dramatically. And so what might be right for you at one point in your life may feel wrong at another. And your doctors and loved ones need to know what to do if you are no longer able to speak for yourself, whether from acute illness or trauma or chronic progressive illness.

I hope that this appendix will put you in the driver's seat of your care. It offers an overall approach to finding the best path through this complex terrain, with specific pointers that are particularly relevant in the setting of the intensive care unit. Starting this process now will empower you to live the life you choose all the way to the very end.

Six Steps Along the Path

The following six steps will start your journey. You should plan to revisit them anytime you have a change in your health status or at least once a year.

1. TAKING STOCK

Although everyone is different, young and healthy bodies are more likely to "spring back" after illness or trauma. As a result, even if they become sick enough to require machines to keep them alive, they may have a better chance of eventually coming off them. But as people age, become ill, or develop dementia, they may decide against keeping their bodies alive at all costs.

What Is Your (or Your Loved One's) Health Status?
- ☐ Young and healthy
- ☐ Older and healthy
- ☐ Chronically ill
- ☐ Serious diagnosis
- ☐ Nearing death

2. UNDERSTANDING THE FUTURE

If you or a loved one has a diagnosed medical illness, it helps to understand the trajectory that is generally associated with it. Dr. Joanne Lynn and co-workers laid out four typical patterns of functional decline before death.

The first pattern describes previously healthy patients who die suddenly from causes like trauma or a surprise heart attack. Such people live at a high level of function until their death.

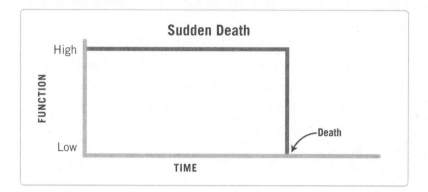

Patients with terminal illnesses, usually in the form of metastatic cancer, can physically function well for a time. But when they begin to deteriorate, as manifested by steady weakening or more hospitalizations, they do so in a fairly linear and unremitting fashion toward death.

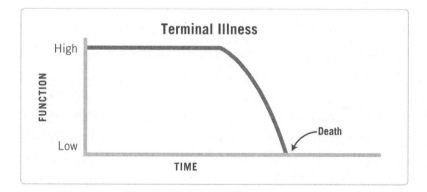

Patients with organ dysfunctions such as emphysema, congestive heart failure, or kidney failure tend to exhibit a trajectory that can be misleading.

When their disease flares up, hospitalization, possibly including a stay in the ICU on life support, might pull them back from the precipice of death. At least temporarily. But with each flare-up, their overall function declines as shown along the graph's vertical axis. And this can be a trap, as patients often believe that we can continue to save them. I see many patients on their fourth or even sixth admission for a heart failure or an emphysema flare-up in as many months. They do not realize that they are approaching their deaths no matter what we do.

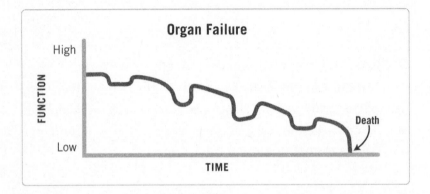

The frailty trajectory, which often co-exists with a diagnosis of dementia, is by far the most common. It applied to 47 percent of the patients in Dr. Lynn's 2002 study. According to the Alzheimer's Association website, one in three seniors dies of Alzheimer's or another dementia. These patients continue to lose function at a steady rate as they approach their deaths.

Understanding these trajectories can help you remain realistic and prepared as you plan for the future. And it can be an excellent jumping-off point for a conversation with your doctor.

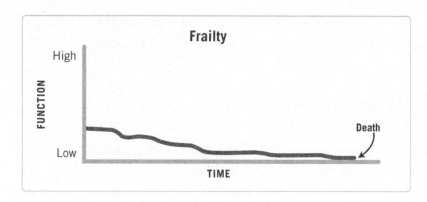

*If You or Your Loved One Has a Diagnosed Illness,
What Is the Likely Health Trajectory?*

☐ Terminal illness
☐ Organ failure
☐ Frailty or dementia
☐ Some combination of the above

3. GETTING SPECIFICS FROM YOUR DOCTOR

Understanding the overall patterns of medical trajectories is help-ful, but you will need to learn more specifics about your, or your loved one's, case from the doctor. What treatments might be of-fered? What are the treatment's potential benefits and burdens? If the benefit is living longer, how much more life can you expect? For burdens, what potential symptoms are you likely to encounter? If you will gain two months but experience severe nausea and vomiting, would it be worth it to you to receive the treatment?

In the following list I've noted conversational strategies for getting this information. You might need to directly ask for the truth for your doctor to give it to you. Consider bringing a trusted friend or family member with you to your appointment to help gather and retain information. And if you are still having trouble communicating with your doctor, you can ask to meet with the palliative care team, whose members have been trained to facilitate these conversations.

Here Are Some Things You Might Say to Your Doctor to Grease the Wheels of Communication:

- Please tell it to me like it is. I want to know what you really think so I can plan.
- You see a lot of patients with [name the disease]. What is the pathway my disease is likely to take?
- Would you be surprised if I were alive in five years? One year? Six months?
- What are the benefits and burdens of the treatment you are suggesting? What are the alternatives? What happens if we don't pursue them?
- What would you choose to do if this were you, your wife, your father?

4. IDENTIFYING WHAT MATTERS

Take some time to write down the things that matter most to you now. How would you rank these principles for yourself? I have drawn from the work of Ezekiel Emanuel to create the following basic checklist to get you started. In the Resources (page 309), I offer further tools for exploring these critical questions.

What Is Your Conception of a Life Worth Living?

- ☐ Every nanosecond counts, no matter my condition.
- ☐ Being free of pain.
- ☐ Having the ability to engage in relationships.
- ☐ Retaining a measure of autonomy (that is, being able to clean myself, think for myself, and get around).
- ☐ Engaging in work or tasks that are meaningful to me.

☐ Being able to live in my own home, or with relatives, as opposed to an institution.

☐ Not being a burden on my family and friends (financially, emotionally, practically, physically).

5. CONSIDERING LIFE PROLONGATION

As an ICU physician, I see many cases where patients' bodies are being kept alive—whether by breathing machines, feeding tubes, dialysis, and/or antibiotics—despite poor prognoses for recovery or return to their previous function. I so often wish that these patients had given some indication to a loved one or a doctor of how they would feel about being kept alive in this condition. Surveys show that almost no one wants that, and yet without a clear opt-out, we doctors feel obligated to keep such patients alive.

If you cannot achieve the lowest quality of life that would be acceptable to you based on your preferences in step 4, where would you fall on this line?

Keep me comfortable and allow me to die naturally ──────────────── Keep me alive at all costs

I assume that many of you will fall toward the left side of this line. But remember, ICU doctors like me will work to keep you alive unless we know for sure.

6. COMMUNICATING AND DOCUMENTING YOUR WISHES

No one can read your mind, including those who love you dearly. You may have the best-laid plans, but if you don't communicate them, chaos can ensue. Even when families are mostly confident that their loved one would not want to be kept alive on machines, removing those machines without a clear directive can simply be too difficult.

There are many helpful tools and online services designed to transmit your wishes to those who need to know—your family, your doctor, and first responders. I will direct you to a few of these in the Resources section. The most basic tool is an Advance Directive (AD). This document serves two major purposes: allowing you to select a surrogate decision maker who will speak for you if you can no longer speak for yourself, and providing a broad sense of your preferences in a few hypothetical medical situations. Please keep in mind that it is not a doctor's order and serves only to provide a general sense of your wishes (see page 78 for a more comprehensive description).

A Do Not Resuscitate (DNR) order is signed by a doctor for a patient in an institution (hospital or nursing home) when it is clear that cardiopulmonary resuscitation is not in line with the patient's preferences. The DNR order is good only for a particular admission at a particular time. If the patient is transferred to another facility, it is rendered void. If you want to remain DNR, make sure to clarify this with your doctor on every admission to any hospital or health care facility, such as a nursing home or a rehabilitation center. And ask your doctor to fill out a Physician Order for Life-Sustaining Treatment (POLST, see below).

A Physician Order for Life-Sustaining Treatment (POLST) follows the patient wherever she goes: home, to another hospital, even across state lines. Like the DNR, the POLST specifies the patient's preferences regarding treatments to be used in the event of cardiopulmonary arrest or other conditions. Unlike the AD, the directives specified in the POLST are legal orders and must be followed by anyone caring for the patient. It is the only form that can release first responders like EMTs, paramedics, and ER

doctors from an obligation to perform the treatments of life prolongation.

The POLST allows you to select between different
approaches—*full treatment,* in which the primary goal is to prolong life using any means necessary (including electric shocks to
the heart and breathing tubes); *comfort-focused treatment,* in which
the primary goal is to maximize comfort and relieve suffering (no
shocks or breathing tubes, but including medicine for pain and
shortness of breath, and oxygen if needed); and a middle category
of *selective treatment,* which includes all strategies for comfort-
focused treatment but also the use of antibiotics, IV fluids, and
masks to try to prolong life while keeping comfort in mind.

The POLST is intended for use by those who are already frail
or seriously ill, where the burden of life-prolonging treatments
may be greater than the benefit. It is particularly important for
those people who are positive they would not want to undergo
certain types of treatment. For those of you who are open to receiving all available treatments, you needn't fill out this form as
they will happen by default. If you do choose to complete a
POLST, you may consider ordering a MedicAlert bracelet as
well. Attached to your body, it is harder to miss than a paper form
(see page 198 for a more comprehensive description).

Still, tools are only tools. They can get lost, damaged, or misinterpreted or simply become outdated. So talk, talk, talk. Create
a living dialogue with your family and with your doctor.

Check the Communication Products That You Feel
Would Be Helpful for You to Complete Right Now:

- ☐ Advance Directive
- ☐ Hospital DNR order
- ☐ POLST form
- ☐ MedicAlert bracelet to supplement your POLST

Avoiding Unnecessary Suffering

I N MY YEARS CARING for seriously ill and dying patients in the ICU, I have noticed a variety of problematic patterns that can arise. The goal of this appendix is to alert you to those situations and provide strategies to mitigate or even avoid them. They fall into two broad areas: physiologic states and treatments/ technology. After describing these factors, I will attempt to address the confusion that I often see regarding the role of hospice and palliative care, which we know from data is an underused resource in the care of patients with serious and end-of-life illness. Please keep in mind that these are very broad, general categories, and I do not intend to advocate for or against any specific treatments. Your case is individual, and I cannot speak to either the particular complications that might arise or the appropriate management strategies.

Physiologic States at the End of Life

Physical Pain • For many, the fear of physical pain is greater than the fear of death. Unfortunately, statistics show that increasing numbers of people are dying in pain, according to their surrogates: 61 percent in 2014, a 12 percent leap from 1998. This despite twenty years of efforts to improve the dying process following the SUPPORT trial of 1996. But data clearly indicate that input from a palliative care team can almost always achieve good pain relief. With its interdisciplinary approach to suffering, palliative care teams are uniquely suited to attend to the physical, spiritual, emotional, and psychological factors so common in the setting of terminal illness. If you or a loved one with serious illness suffers from physical pain that is limiting your quality of life, I recommend asking for a palliative care consultation.

Shortness of Breath • The lungs can be compromised by a variety of diseases, including cancers, pneumonia, emphysema, and heart failure. If not well managed, the resulting shortness of breath can be terrifying and profoundly impact a person's quality of life, and death. If the primary team is having trouble managing shortness of breath, the palliative care service or, if appropriate, hospice should be called in, as both are adept at managing this serious symptom, not only acutely but over the long term.

Hemorrhage • Cancers and other tissue inflammations can cause rapid internal bleeding if large blood vessels are eroded. Patients may in fact die from hemorrhaging that cannot be stopped. Sometimes the bleeding is invisible to us, remaining within the abdominal or chest cavity, but other times the blood will exit the body, through either the mouth or nose, or from below. This can be very frightening and cause profound trauma for loved ones.

But such hemorrhage can be anticipated and managed well, even in the home, particularly by hospice services. Your physician will know if there is such a risk. If this is the case, I suggest you discuss with your doctor the possibility of involving hospice in your care.

Bowel Obstruction • Many diseases, particularly cancers, can result in partial or full bowel obstructions, which impact the passage of food through the intestinal tract. This may cause serious nausea, vomiting, and painful bloating. There are many treatments to try, but sometimes the obstruction simply cannot be bypassed. In this case, feeding by mouth or through a feeding tube will generally not benefit the patient and may worsen symptoms. This can be emotionally devastating, especially when patients remain alert and awake. For refractory cases, talk to your doctor about the possibility of a venting gastrostomy tube.

Treatment and Technology at the End of Life

Palliative (also Called Compassionate) Extubation • It is not infrequent that surrogate decision makers decide to withdraw a breathing tube from a dying patient. What happens next can vary greatly from patient to patient. Some pass away within minutes, others in days to weeks. Some appear calm and asymptomatic, while others manifest disturbing clinical signs. In my experience, families who are prepared for all eventualities do better than those who aren't. Here are a couple of things to keep in mind.

You may hear a lot of harsh noises coming from your loved one's mouth after the tube comes out. It can sound like the patient is struggling to breathe, but most of the time it is just part of the dying process. This is a common and expected occurrence, usually the result of laxity of the throat muscles. Rarely is it a more serious obstruction, but your doctor should nonetheless be monitoring this process to ensure that there is no unnecessary distress.

Most likely the feeding tube was removed at the same time as the breathing tube. In cases where patients live longer than expected, I have seen some families grow panicked at the thought that their loved one is not being fed. While these are understandable human emotions, it is important to remember that feeding a dying body will likely inflict discomfort and can even be dangerous.

Chemotherapy in Terminal Cancer • "Palliative chemotherapy" is commonly used in patients with previously treated organ cancers whose life expectancy is less than six months. The intention is not to cure but to prolong their lives and improve symptoms. However, several recent studies indicate that these patients should not receive chemotherapy at all. These studies show that chemotherapy at this point not only worsens the quality of life before death, it also puts patients at increased risk of highly mechanized deaths in the ICU. This applies especially to those who are young or still have a good functional status, who ultimately may have the most to lose. Yet doctors continue to prescribe it, often without discussing the poor prognosis with the patient. If you or your loved one has been offered "palliative chemotherapy" for cancer that has spread and already been treated, make sure that you sit down with your doctor to clarify your life expectancy. If it is less than six months, regardless of your current functional status, the latest studies recommend against receiving chemotherapy. As Dr. Charles Blanke, an oncologist, and Dr. Erik Fromme, a palliative care physician, state in an editorial accompanying the publication of one study: "If an oncologist suspects the death of a patient in the next 6 months, the default should be no active treatment. Let us help patients with metastatic cancer make good decisions at this sad, but often inevitable, stage. Let us not contribute to the suffering that cancer, and often associated therapy, brings, particularly at the end."

Implantable Cardioverter Defibrillators (ICDs) • Increasing numbers of patients are receiving implantable cardioverter defibrillators, which shock arrhythmic hearts back into a normal rhythm in order to prevent sudden death. These devices have saved countless lives that would otherwise have been lost. There is some psychological distress caused by the pain and unpredictable timing of these shocks, but life prolongation is often worth the burden. However, as patients with these implanted devices approach the end of their lives, a problem can arise. When their heart rhythm becomes unstable, they will be shocked, even in the minutes before death. Possibly repeatedly. And so it is imperative that people with such devices determine if and when they want to have them turned off, allowing for a sudden, painless death at the next occurrence. This deactivation is done easily and non-invasively by a physician using a special machine. Unfortunately, while almost all doctors surveyed agree that deactivation is appropriate in terminally ill patients, these conversations happen only 27 percent of the time. And even for patients with ICDs who are DNR, for whom death is already expected imminently, the conversations are happening less than 50 percent of the time. If you or your loved one has such a device, make sure that you are cognizant of this risk and discuss it with your physician.

Feeding Tubes and Dementia • Dementia is a disease with a predictable trajectory, and one of the eventual complications is that a person loses his ability to swallow safely. Many patients with dementia end up in the ICU on breathing machines with pneumonias contracted by aspirating food or gastric contents. Often, if a patient survives, a decision is made to insert a feeding tube directly into the stomach in order to bypass the dysfunctional swallowing mechanism. But there is a lot of evidence to suggest that these tubes can actually make things worse for a patient. Many, including the American Geriatrics Society, advocate that patients with end-stage dementia receive careful hand-feeding instead of using a feeding tube. In many hospitals, there is no discussion about this complex issue, and the assumption is that everyone would want a feeding tube. And doctors and patients alike can forget that the artificial nutrition that comes through this tube is not food but a medical therapy that can be refused like any other treatment.

Voluntary Stopping of Eating and Drinking (VSED) • Although a rare occurrence, some terminally ill patients with intact mental functioning choose to hasten their deaths by ceasing to eat and drink. Often this is due to the person's perception that her quality of life is no longer acceptable. The act may also provide a sense of control and autonomy at this most vulnerable time of life.

Stopping or Starting Dialysis • The kidneys are responsible for cleaning the blood, a critical process for sustaining life. If they are no longer functioning, dialysis machines can be used to filter and clean a person's blood, typically several times a week, siphoning it out of and into the patient's body through a catheter or surgically enlarged blood vessel. Many patients whose kidneys have failed are able to live for years thanks to ongoing dialysis. But as they begin to approach the ends of their lives, there may come a time to stop using this technology that had previously been so beneficial. Dialysis usually requires travel to a special center three times per week. Patients must sit for hours as their blood is run through the machine and cleaned. In addition to this requirement, dialysis is not a perfect substitute for functioning kidneys, and dialysis over years takes its toll. Patients lose weight, frequently feel nausea and fatigue, and gradually weaken. And so the burdens of this treatment in a patient whose body is now dying—whether from chronic kidney disease or a process like cancer—may become too great. But the habit of dialysis can be hard to break. It may have become a part of a person's life, and the idea of stopping it, even if its burdens are outweighing its benefits, might be overwhelming. This too is something that is worth discussing with your doctor.

For those patients with kidneys that are failing due to critical illness rather than a chronic condition as above, dialysis may be offered in the hospital or ICU environment. If you or a loved one develops kidney failure abruptly, or even over days, make sure that you learn more about the underlying condition that caused the kidneys to fail. Some people feel that if they are actively dying from an untreatable condition like cancer, then prolonging life through dialysis would not achieve their goals. Others feel that any treatment that prolongs life would be worth trying. Ultimately, it's up to the patient or surrogate to weigh the benefits and burdens and decide.

Extracorporeal Membrane Oxygenation (ECMO) • Where dialysis cleans blood in the place of failed kidneys, ECMO is a developing technology that can oxygenate blood in the place of failed lungs and/or hearts. The intended use of this technology is to keep a patient alive until he recovers from an acute illness such as severe influenza ("bridge to recovery") or can receive an organ transplant ("bridge to transplant"). In short, it is intended as a bridge to health, not a long-term solution. Unlike dialysis, which only requires three touchpoints with the medical system per week, ECMO machinery currently requires the patient to live in the ICU. With the rising use of this technology, there have been increasing numbers of cases where it becomes clear that a patient, stabilized and alert on ECMO, will never be able to live independent of the machine, either because the organ will not recover as previously hoped or a transplant is deemed not feasible. The patient will then remain in limbo, tethered to these machines in the ICU. For most of us, this would not be an acceptable quality of life, but once a person arrives at that place, it is very hard to terminate the treatment keeping her alive. This is something to keep in mind if this treatment is offered: What would you do if ECMO turned into a destination therapy for you or your loved one, as opposed to a bridge to recovery?

Palliation at the End of Life

Understanding the Landscape: The Difference Between Hospice and Palliative Care • Palliative care attends to the needs of patients with serious symptoms, whether physical, psychological, spiritual, or emotional. It is usually delivered to patients in the hospital or in an outpatient clinic. Practitioners are trained to manage these symptoms as well as to communicate information and coordinate understanding among all relevant parties. Palliative care is appropriate for anyone who has symptom management and communication needs from serious illness, not simply those who are approaching death.

Hospice services provide palliative care for terminally ill patients who may have only months to live. These services are only available to patients who are no longer receiving curative treatment for their underlying disease. Hospice services are usually delivered in the home but can also be provided in nursing homes.

Palliative Options for Patients Desiring Continued Disease-Focused Treatment • For progressive diseases such as cancer, congestive heart failure, progressive neurologic dysfunction (such as Lou Gehrig's disease), emphysema, and others, there is a benefit to including palliative care for management of symptoms while continuing to treat the underlying disease.

Cancer is a good example of this. In 2012, the American Society of Clinical Oncology recommended that "combined standard oncology care and palliative care should be considered early in the course of illness for any patient with metastatic cancer or high symptom burden." Over the ensuing years, evidence has accumulated to show that palliative care is an excellent complementary therapy for many cancer patients, even in early-stage cancers or cases in which cure is expected. Concurrent palliative care decreased symptom burden, increased patient satisfaction, lowered chance of dying in the ICU and on breathing machines, and reduced the burden on family and caregivers. Some studies have shown that palliative care provided alongside cancer care actually prolonged survival.

Unfortunately, there are serious barriers to combining these two modalities of care, both on the doctor and on the patient side. Oncologists and other specialists may feel that they can provide palliative treatments to their patients themselves and only consult the palliative care specialty services when patients are imminently dying with intractable symptoms. And so much of its potential benefit is missed. And patients might associate the term "palliative" with end-stage care and not be open to trying it.

Moreover, for chemotherapy patients living at home, receiving palliative care requires going to a clinic appointment, which is difficult when a patient is weak and tired. Unfortunately, at the time of this writing, palliative care in the home (also called hospice) is not available to those continuing to receive cancer-focused treatment. Yet data are clear that many cancer patients benefit significantly from hospice services, certainly with improvements in quality of life but also with life prolongation in several types of cancer. If you carry a prognosis of six months or less, this is something to take into serious consideration as you weigh the benefits and burdens of the treatments offered to you. In short, I would recommend that for those patients with cancer that has spread to other parts of the body and who have not responded well to chemotherapy, it might be time to switch to hospice.

A Note on "Right to Die" Legislation

Several states now have Physician Aid in Dying (PAD) laws, which enable patients to request lethal drugs from their physicians in order to end their lives. This is not euthanasia—illegal in the United States—in which physicians administer the lethal dose to the patient. PAD laws require the patient to be physically able to administer the dose to themselves. These laws require patients to carry a diagnosis of terminal illness, with a prognosis of less than six months. Oregon's law has been in effect since 1997. In the fifteen years between 1997 and 2012, a total of 673 patients chose to exercise this right. This has been a polarizing issue for many, with some feeling that this is an essential right and others questioning whether such laws put vulnerable people at risk.

While this topic generates considerable controversy, in my experience it potentially applies to a tiny segment of the population. My hope is that it is used only as a last resort for patients for whom everything else, including excellent palliative care, has been tried.

Resources

THE FOLLOWING LIST OF websites are those I believe will be helpful to you on your journey. This is by no means an exhaustive list but rather a tour of the types of resources that are out there.

1. Considering and Communicating Personal Preferences

Prepare (prepareforyourcare.org) Uses videos of people thinking about their end-of-life preferences to walk you through the steps of choosing a surrogate decision maker, determining your own preferences, and communicating these preferences. It functions as an online coach and motivates you to get started on the process.
The Conversation Project (theconversationproject.org) Their starter kit and other tools are dedicated to helping people begin the conversation with friends and families about their end-of-life wishes.

Go Wish Card Game (gowish.org) Gives you an easy, even enter-taining way to talk about what's most important to you with your family and friends.

Death Cafe (deathcafe.com) Coffee gatherings of people, often strangers, at a variety of coffee shops and yogurt bars in your area, with a downloadable guide to the conversation.

Death over Dinner (deathoverdinner.org) Organized dinners for groups of people, with prompts and materials provided to en-courage and facilitate deep communication and conversation.

2. Documenting Your Preferences

POLST (polst.org) Provides state-specific POLST forms.

Five Wishes (agingwithdignity.org/five-wishes) This form func-tions as an Advance Directive in most states but uses more ordi-nary language and focuses more on personal and spiritual priorities.

Advance Directive forms (caringinfo.org) State-specific AD forms.

My Directives (mydirectives.com) Helps you create an Advance Di-rective that can be emailed to your doctor and family.

3. Helpful Websites

Jessica Nutik Zitter, MD (jessicazitter.com) This is my own web-site, which contains links to my writing and talks on these topics. There is also a resource page with a regularly updated list of tools and sites for your use.

Get Palliative Care (getpalliativecare.org) This site offers a com-prehensive guide to the benefits of palliative care medicine.

National Hospice and Palliative Care Organization (caringinfo .org) This website offers guidance to those dealing with serious illness, including advice on advance care planning, grieving, and caregiving.

NHDD *(nhdd.org/public-resources)* This site, from National Health-care Decisions Day, offers a wide range of links and resources to encourage and support advance care planning.

FOR HEALTH CARE PROVIDERS AND INSTITUTIONS

ACP *(acpdecisions.org)* Video library of decision aids that help patients and their clinicians discuss difficult topics in a neutral fashion.

VitalTalk *(vitaltalk.org)* Teaches clinicians to communicate with their patients more skillfully and honestly about difficult topics.

Lown Institute *(lowninstitute.org)* An organization that promotes patient-centered approaches to health care.

Ariadne Labs *(ariadnelabs.org)* Provides guidance for clinicians to initiate conversations about serious illness.

Center to Advance Palliative Care *(capc.org)* Resource for hospitals and other health care settings interested in developing palliative care programs.

Notes

CHAPTER ONE: ALONE IN THE TRENCHES

PAGE 7: **"Hashem [God] will remove from you every illness":** *Chumash, The Stone Edition,* Rabbis Nosson Scherman and Meir Zlotowitz (Brooklyn, New York: Mesorah Publications, Ltd., 2000).

PAGE 7: **"Whoever saves a life, it is considered as if he saved an entire world":** Mishnah Sanhedrin 4:9; Yerushalmi Talmud, Tractate Sanhedrin 37a.

PAGE 8: **"he who asks questions sheds blood":** Shulhan Arukh, Orah Hayyim 328:2.

PAGE 8: **imposed a 10 percent quota on Jewish students beginning in 1920 that lasted until the 1960s:** Gerald Tulchinsky, *Canada's Jews* (Toronto: University of Toronto Press, 2008), p. 415.

CHAPTER TWO: THE END-OF-LIFE CONVEYOR BELT

PAGE 25: **They cost as much as the average home in 1930:** Smithsonian National Museum of American History, Behring Center, "The Iron Lung and Other Equipment," available at amhistory.si.edu/polio/howpolio/ironlung.htm.

PAGE 25: **these metal boxes kept many thousands of people alive:** Daniel J. Wilson, "Braces, Wheelchairs, and Iron Lungs: The Paralyzed Body and the Machinery of Rehabilitation in the Polio Epidemics," *Journal of Medical Humanities* 26, nos. 2–3 (2005): 173–90.

PAGE 26: **Our country houses many more ICU beds per capita than other comparable nations:** R. A. Gooch, "ICU Bed Supply, Utilization, and Health Care Spending," *Journal of the American Medical Association* 311, no. 6 (2014): 567–68.

PAGE 33: **Graduating medical students have been reciting the oath of Hippocrates for the past five hundred years:** Raphael Hulkower, "The History of the Hippocratic Oath: Outdated, Inauthentic, and Yet Still Relevant," *Einstein Journal of Biology and Medicine* 25, no. 1 (2010): 41–44.

PAGE 33: **"I will remember [...] that there is art to medicine as well as science, and that warmth, sympathy, and understanding may outweigh the surgeon's knife or the chemist's drug":** Peter Tyson, "The Hippocratic Oath Today: Hippocratic Oath: Modern Version," March 27, 2001, available at pbs.org/wgbh/nova/body/hippocratic-oath -today.html.

PAGE 35: **the catheter was routinely being inserted in 20 to 40 percent of all ICU patients:** Renda Soylemez Wiener and H. Gilbert Welch, "Trends in the Use of the Pulmonary Artery Catheter in the United States, 1993–2004," *Journal of the American Medical Association* 298, no. 4 (2007): 423–29.

PAGE 35: **annual costs for the procedure exceeded $2 billion:** James E. Dalen, "The Pulmonary Artery Catheter—Friend, Foe, or Accomplice?," *Journal of the American Medical Association* 286, no. 3 (2001): 348–50.

PAGE 36: **published in the reputable *Journal of the American Medical Association*, and there was no ignoring it:** Alfred F. Connors, Theodore Speroff, Neal V. Dawson, et al., "The Effectiveness of Right Heart Catheterization in the Initial Care of Critically Ill Patients," *Journal of the American Medical Association* 276, no. 11 (1996): 889–97.

PAGE 36: **the numbers we assiduously pulled from the catheter to guide our treatment plan were fool's gold:** Vinay K. Dhingra, John C. Fenwick, Keith R. Walley, et al., "Lack of Agreement between Thermodilution and Fick Cardiac Output in Critically Ill Patients," *Chest Journal* 122, no. 3 (2002): 990–97; and Paul E. Marik, "Obituary: Pulmonary Artery Catheter 1970 to 2013," *Annals of Intensive Care* 3, no. 1 (2013): 38.

PAGE 36: **the Swan actually increased the odds of death by 24 percent:** Connors et al., "The Effectiveness of Right Heart Catheterization."

PAGE 36: **A firestorm raged in the medical literature for years afterward:** Neill Soni, "Swan Song for the Swan-Ganz Catheter?," *British Medical Journal* 313, no. 7060 (1996): 763; and Max Harry Weil, "The Assault on the Swan-Ganz Catheter: A Case History of Constrained Technology, Constrained Bedside Clinicians, and Constrained Monetary Expenditures," *Chest Journal* 113, no. 5 (1998): 1379–86.

PAGE 37: **SUPPORT was designed as a two-phase study:** Alfred F. Connors, Neal V. Dawson, Norman A. Desbiens, et al., "A Controlled Trial to Improve Care for Seriously Ill Hospitalized Patients: The Study to Understand Prognoses and Preferences for Outcomes and Risks of Treatments (SUPPORT)," *Journal of the American Medical Association* 274, no. 20 (1995): 1591–98.

PAGE 39: **"It is inconceivable for me to manage a critically ill patient with a heart that's not working well without this instrument":** R. Winslow, "Study Questions Safety, Cost of Catheter Device for Heart," *Wall Street Journal*, September 18, 1996.

PAGE 43: **in 1999, Promoting Excellence decided to go right to the belly of the beast, the ICU:** Ira Byock, "Improving Palliative Care in Intensive Care Units: Identifying Strategies and Interventions That Work," *Critical Care Medicine* 34, no. 11 (2006): S302–5.

PAGE 43: **only four institutions were awarded grants, which they received in March 2003:** American Association of Critical-Care Nurses, "Promoting Palliative Care Excellence in Intensive Care Demonstration Projects," available at aacn.org/wd/palliative/content/grantees.pcms?menu =practice.

PAGE 50: **multiple studies have shown that providing patients with analgesia does not compromise diagnosis:** Carlos Manterola, Manuel Vial, Javier Moraga, and Paula Astudillo, "Analgesia in Patients with Acute Abdominal Pain," *Cochrane Database of Systematic Reviews* 1, no. 1 (2011): 1–33.

PAGE 50: **Over 50 percent of Americans die in pain:** Adam E. Singer, Daniella Meeker, Joan M. Teno, et al., "Symptom Trends in the Last Year of Life from 1998 to 2010: A Cohort Study," *Annals of Internal Medicine* 162, no. 3 (2015): 175–83.

PAGE 50: **Seventy percent die in institutions:** National Center for Health Statistics, "National Vital Statistics System: Deaths by Place of Death, Age, Race, and Sex: United States 1999–2005," Table GMWK309, Cen-

[314]   NOTES

ters for Disease Control and Prevention, available at cdc.gov/nchs/nvss /mortality/gmwk309.htm.

PAGE 50: **30 percent of families lose most of their life savings while caring for a dying loved one:** Kenneth E. Covinsky, Lee Goldman, E. Francis Cook, et al., "The Impact of Serious Illness on Patients' Families," *Journal of the American Medical Association* 272, no. 23 (1994): 1839–44.

PAGE 50: **choosing hospice over continued disease-oriented treatment prolonged the lives of patients with several types of life-limiting diseases by an average of a month:** S. R. Connor, Bruce Pyenson, Kathryn Fitch, et al., "Comparing Hospice and Nonhospice Patient Survival among Patients Who Die within a Three-Year Window," *Journal of Pain and Symptom Management* 33, no. 3 (2007): 238.

PAGE 50: **patients with serious cancers receiving palliative care consultations in addition to standard care lived longer by an average of two months:** Jennifer S. Temel, Joseph A. Greer, Alona Muzikansky, et al., "Early Palliative Care for Patients with Metastatic Non–Small-Cell Lung Cancer," *New England Journal of Medicine* 363, no. 8 (2010): 733–42.

CHAPTER THREE: ABANDONED IN A SEA OF OPTIONS

PAGE 66: **American patients dying of cancer had twice as many ICU days as similar patients from the other countries studied:** Justin E. Bekelman, Scott D. Halpern, Carl Rudolf Blankart, et al., "Comparison of Site of Death, Health Care Utilization, and Hospital Expenditures for Patients Dying with Cancer in 7 Developed Countries," *Journal of the American Medical Association* 315, no. 3 (2016): 272–83.

PAGE 68: **While only 9 percent of students entering medical school in 1965 were women, by 1975, that number was over 20 percent; today, it approaches 50 percent:** Diana M. Lautenberger, Valerie M. Dandar, Claudia L. Raezer, and Rae Anne Sloane, "The State of Women in Academic Medicine: The Pipeline and Pathways to Leadership, 2013–2014," Association of American Medical Colleges, 2014, Table 1, available at aamc.org/members/gwims/statistics.

PAGE 68: **And in 1972, the world learned about the egregious experiments at Tuskegee University:** Jean Heller, "Syphilis Victims in U.S. Study Went Untreated for 40 Years," *The New York Times*, July 26, 1972.

PAGE 73: **hospice services . . . are not available to those receiving disease-focused treatments such as chemotherapy:** David J. Casarett and Timothy E. Quill, "'I'm Not Ready for Hospice': Strategies for Timely and Effective Hospice Discussions," *Annals of Internal Medicine* 146, no. 6 (2007): 443–49.

PAGE 74: **patients on breathing machines demonstrated that the better the quality of clinician–family communication, the less life support was elected:** Alyssa Majesko, Seo Yeon Hong, Lisa Weissfeld, and Douglas B. White, "Identifying Family Members Who May Struggle in the Role of Surrogate Decision Maker," *Critical Care Medicine* 40, no. 8 (2012): 2281.

PAGE 74: **Another study showed that people were less likely to want CPR after they learned what it actually entailed:** Donald J. Murphy, David Burrows, Sara Santilli, et al., "The Influence of the Probability of Survival on Patients' Preferences Regarding Cardiopulmonary Resuscitation," *New England Journal of Medicine* 330, no. 8 (1994): 545–49.

PAGE 80: **the "thirty-day mortality statistic":** New York State Department of Health, "Percutaneous Coronary Intervention (PCI) in New York State: 2008–2010," August 2012, available at health.ny.gov/statistics /diseases/cardiovascular/docs/pci_2008-2010.pdf.

PAGE 81: **worrying reports of surgical patients dying slowly for weeks after their surgeries, for whom a palliative care consultation was delayed until day thirty-one post-op:** Paula Span, "A Surgery Standard under Fire," *The New York Times*, March 2, 2015.

PAGE 86: **CPR is often of no real benefit for many of the patients upon whom we use it:** Graham Nichol, Brian Leroux, Henry Wang, et al., "Trial of Continuous or Interrupted Chest Compressions during CPR," *New England Journal of Medicine* 373, no. 23 (2015): 2203–14.

PAGE 86: **feeding tubes can actually be harmful for many:** Clinical Practice and Models of Care Committee, "American Geriatrics Society Feeding Tubes in Advanced Dementia Position Statement," *Journal of the American Geriatrics Society* 62, no. 8 (2014): 1590.

PAGE 86: **these facts are widely unknown, even by some of the physicians who administer these procedures:** Kerin Jones, Manish Garg, Doru Bali, et al., "The Knowledge and Perceptions of Medical Personnel Relating to Outcome after Cardiac Arrest," *Resuscitation* 69, no. 2 (2006): 235–39.

PAGE 96: **The data are grim:** Jeremy M. Kahn, Nicole M. Benson, Dina Appleby, et al., "Long-Term Acute Care Hospital Utilization after Critical Illness," *Journal of the American Medical Association* 303, no. 22 (2010): 2253–59.

PAGE 96: **as of 2010, there were more than 100,000 chronically ventilated patients in the United States:** Judith E. Nelson, Christopher E.

Cox, Aluko A. Hope, and Shannon S. Carson, "Chronic Critical Illness," *American Journal of Respiratory and Critical Care Medicine* 182, no. 4 (2010): 446–54.

PAGE 96: **But the most disturbing study I saw was a survey of physicians and caregivers predicting the outcomes of 126 patients at the time of tracheostomy placement:** Christopher E. Cox, Tereza Martinu, Shailaja J. Sathy, et al., "Expectations and Outcomes of Prolonged Mechanical Ventilation," *Critical Care Medicine* 37, no. 11 (2009): 2888.

PAGE 99: **In 2011, Ken Murray, a retired family practitioner in Los Angeles, wrote an opinion piece that went viral:** Ken Murray, "How Doctors Die: It's Not Like the Rest of Us, but It Should Be," *Zocolo Public Square,* November 30, 2011. http://www.zocalopublicsquare.org/2011/11/30 /how-doctors-die/ideas/nexus/.

PAGE 99: **Nearly nine in ten said they would choose a do-not-resuscitate status near the end of life:** Vyjeyanthi S. Periyakoil, Eric Neri, Ann Fong, and Helena Kraemer, "Do unto Others: Doctors' Personal End-of-Life Resuscitation Preferences and Their Attitudes toward Advance Directives," *PLOS ONE* 9, no. 5 (2014): e98246.

PAGE 99: **Physicians were less likely to die in a hospital or other health care facility than was the general population:** Saul Blecker, Norman J. Johnson, Sean Altekruse, and Leora I. Horwitz, "Association of Occupation as a Physician with Likelihood of Dying in a Hospital," *Journal of the American Medical Association* 315, no. 3 (2016): 301–3.

PAGE 99: **and doctors received significantly less intensive care before death:** Joel S. Weissman, Zara Cooper, Joseph A. Hyder, et al., "End-of-Life Care Intensity for Physicians, Lawyers, and the General Population," *Journal of the American Medical Association* 315, no. 3 (2016): 303–5.

PAGE 100: **This practice for patients with progressive metastatic cancers is coming under scrutiny for not being of benefit and in fact causing harm:** Holly G. Prigerson, Yuhua Bao, Manish A. Shah, et al., "Chemotherapy Use, Performance Status, and Quality of Life at the End of Life," *JAMA Oncology* 1, no. 6 (2015): 778–84.

PAGE 101: **Diane Meier, a palliative care physician at The Mount Sinai Hospital in New York, speaks to the other side of that equation:** Diane E. Meier, "'I Don't Want Jenny to Think I'm Abandoning Her': Views on Overtreatment," *Health Affairs* 33, no. 5 (2014): 895–98.

PAGE 106: **In an editorial in the** *New England Journal of Medicine*, **David Casarett discusses the "therapeutic illusion":** David Casarett, "The Science of Choosing Wisely—Overcoming the Therapeutic Illusion," *New England Journal of Medicine* 374, no. 13 (2016): 1203–5.

PAGE 107: **One study published in the** *British Medical Journal* **in 2000 demonstrated that physicians overestimate their patients' duration of remaining life by 5.3-fold:** Nicholas A. Christakis, Julia L. Smith, Colin Murray Parkes, and Elizabeth B. Lamont, "Extent and Determinants of Error in Doctors' Prognoses in Terminally Ill Patients: Prospective Cohort Study," *British Medical Journal* 320, no. 7233 (2000): 469–73.

PAGE 107: **patients are more likely to learn realistic information about their disease trajectory and prognosis while in their doctor's waiting room than during the actual office encounter:** Sarah Elizabeth Harrington and Thomas J. Smith, "The Role of Chemotherapy at the End of Life: 'When Is Enough, Enough?,'" *Journal of the American Medical Association* 299, no. 22 (2008): 2667–78.

PAGE 131: **while surrogates clearly accepted optimistic prognoses and understood their implications, they tended to discount or even disagree with pessimistic prognoses from doctors:** Lucas S. Zier, Peter D. Sottile, Seo Yeon Hong, et al., "Surrogate Decision Makers' Interpretation of Prognostic Information: A Mixed-Methods Study," *Annals of Internal Medicine* 156, no. 5 (2012): 360–66.

PAGE 131: **A recent study in** *JAMA Oncology*: Kimberson Tanco, Wadih Rhondali, Pedro Perez-Cruz, et al., "Patient Perception of Physician Compassion after a More Optimistic vs a Less Optimistic Message," *JAMA Oncology* 1, no. 2 (2015): 176–83.

PAGE 139: **which the American Society of Clinical Oncology recommends as standard protocol for anybody with metastatic cancer and/or a high symptom burden:** Thomas J. Smith, Sarah Temin, Erin R. Alesi, et al., "American Society of Clinical Oncology Provisional Clinical Opinion: The Integration of Palliative Care into Standard Oncology Care," *Journal of Clinical Oncology* 30, no. 8 (2012): 880–87.

PAGE 140: **excellent palliative care live on average two months longer than those who continue disease-directed treatments alone:** Jennifer S. Temel, Joseph A. Greer, Alona Muzikansky, et al., "Early Palliative Care for Patients with Metastatic Non–Small-Cell Lung Cancer," *New England Journal of Medicine* 363, no. 8 (2010): 733–42.

PAGE 143: **"You have to understand . . . A family meeting is a proce-**

dure, and it requires no less skill than performing an operation": Atul Gawande, *Being Mortal: Illness, Medicine, and What Matters Most at the End of Life* (New York: Metropolitan Books, 2014), p. 181.

CHAPTER FIVE: WHERE WE COME FROM

PAGE 150: **African Americans tend to die differently from whites, receiving more aggressive treatment without benefit at the end of life:** Howard B. Degenholtz, Stephen B. Thomas, and Michael J. Miller, "Race and the Intensive Care Unit: Disparities and Preferences for End-of-Life Care," *Critical Care Medicine* 31, no. 5 (2003): S373–78; and Firas Abdollah, Jesse D. Sammon, Kaustav Majumder, et al., "Racial Disparities in End-of-Life Care among Patients with Prostate Cancer: A Population-Based Study," *Journal of the National Comprehensive Cancer Network* 13, no. 9 (2015): 1131–38.

PAGE 150: **and experiencing more uncontrolled symptoms:** Karen O. Anderson, Carmen R. Green, and Richard Payne, "Racial and Ethnic Disparities in Pain: Causes and Consequences of Unequal Care," *Journal of Pain* 10, no. 12 (2009): 1187–204.

PAGE 150: **They are also 40 percent more likely to die in a hospital than their white counterparts:** Andrea Gruneir, Vincent Mor, Sherry Weitzen, et al., "Where People Die: A Multilevel Approach to Understanding Influences on Site of Death in America," *Medical Care Research and Review* 64, no. 4 (2007): 351–78.

PAGE 150: **and much less likely to enroll in hospice:** Robert L. Ludke and Douglas R. Smucker, "Racial Differences in the Willingness to Use Hospice Services," *Journal of Palliative Medicine* 10, no. 6 (2007): 1329–37.

PAGE 150: **or complete Advance Directives:** Kimberly S. Johnson, "Racial and Ethnic Disparities in Palliative Care," *Journal of Palliative Medicine* 16, no. 11 (2013): 1329–34.

PAGE 150: **The 2013 Pew Research study on end-of-life preferences:** Pew Research Center, "Views on End of Life Medical Treatments: Growing Minority of Americans Say Doctors Should Do Everything Possible to Keep Them Alive," November 21, 2013, available at pewforum.org/2013/11/21/views-on-end-of-life-medical-treatments/#personal-wishes.

PAGE 154: **broad categories: individualist (North America and northern Europe) and collectivist (Asia and southern Europe):** Tatsuya Morita, Yasuhiro Oyama, Shao-Yi Cheng, et al., "Palliative Care Physicians' Attitudes toward Patient Autonomy and a Good Death in East Asian Countries," *Journal of Pain and Symptom Management* 50, no. 2 (2015): 190–99.

PAGE 154: **In a 2000 study comparing attitudes on patient autonomy between physicians in Japan and those in the United States:** Gregory W. Ruhnke, Sandra R. Wilson, Takashi Akamatsu, et al., "Ethical Decision Making and Patient Autonomy: A Comparison of Physicians and Patients in Japan and the United States," *Chest Journal* 118, no. 4 (2000): 1172–82.

PAGE 155: **in 2015, after palliative care had penetrated further into Japan's society, that number rose to 82 percent:** Morita et al., "Palliative Care Physicians' Attitudes toward Patient Autonomy," p. 190.

PAGE 156: **It is no surprise that patients receive safer and more satisfactory care when they are provided with professional language services:** Leah S. Karliner, Elizabeth A. Jacobs, Alice Chen, and Sunita Mutha, "Do Professional Interpreters Improve Clinical Care for Patients with Limited English Proficiency? A Systematic Review of the Literature," *Health Services Research* 42, no. 2 (2007): 727–54.

CHAPTER SIX: WHO WE ARE

PAGE 186: **"All happy families are alike; each unhappy family is unhappy in its own way":** Leo Tolstoy, *Anna Karenina: A Novel in Eight Parts*, trans. Richard Pevear and Larissa Volokhonsky (New York: Penguin Books, 2002).

PAGE 198: **A 2015 study in *JAMA* Surgery:** Peter J. Kneuertz, George J. Chang, Chung-Yuan Hu, et al., "Overtreatment of Young Adults with Colon Cancer: More Intense Treatments with Unmatched Survival Gains," *JAMA Surgery* 150, no. 5 (2015): 402–9.

PAGE 201: **Bisphosphonates had less than a 1 percent risk of complications:** Salvatore L. Ruggiero, Thomas B. Dodson, John Fantasia, et al., "American Association of Oral and Maxillofacial Surgeons Position Paper on Medication-Related Osteonecrosis of the Jaw—2014 Update," *Journal of Oral and Maxillofacial Surgery* 72, no. 10 (2014): 1938–56.

PAGE 205: **Checkbox A: Choice Not to Prolong Life:** "Advanced Healthcare Directive Form," http://oag.ca.gov/sites/all/files/agweb/pdfs/consumers/Probate CodeAdvancedHealthCareDirectiveForm-fillable.pdf.

CHAPTER SEVEN: THE PERSONAL TOLL

PAGE 218: **It has been found to be alarmingly prevalent in doctors compared to the general population. Its impacts, which include high rates of depression and compassion fatigue, are severe for both the doctor and her patients:** Tait D. Shanafelt, Sonja Boone,

Litjen Tan, et al., "Burnout and Satisfaction with Work-Life Balance among US Physicians Relative to the General US Population," *Archives of Internal Medicine* 172, no. 18 (2012): 1377–85.

PAGE 218: **Palliative care is one of the lowest-paid specialties, with a median compensation of $215,000 per year, while a dermatologist who performs specialized skin cancer surgery makes over $700,000:** Cortney Petersheim, "Physician Compensation Report," Resolve Physician Agency, October 4, 2015, available at resolvephysicianagency.com/career/average-physician-salary.

PAGE 220: **The acknowledgment of the unique stressors of palliative care physicians is a very recent phenomenon:** Giselle K. Perez, Vivian Haime, Vicki Jackson, et al., "Promoting Resiliency among Palliative Care Clinicians: Stressors, Coping Strategies, and Training Needs," *Journal of Palliative Medicine* 18, no. 4 (2015): 332–37.

PAGE 222: **moral distress was first defined by Andrew Jameton in the nursing literature in 1984:** Andrew Jameton, *Nursing Practice: The Ethical Issues* (Englewood Cliffs, NJ: Prentice Hall, 1984).

PAGE 222: **"perceived violation of one's core values and duties":** Elizabeth Gingell Epstein and Ann Baile Hamric, "Moral Distress, Moral Residue, and the Crescendo Effect," *Journal of Clinical Ethics* 20, no. 4 (2009): 330.

PAGE 222: **responsible for major problems among health care providers, including feelings of guilt, anger, and self-blame, as well as anxiety and depression:** ibid.

PAGE 222: **burnout and compassion fatigue have also been attributed to moral distress:** Virginia M. Mason, Gail Leslie, Kathleen Clark, et al., "Compassion Fatigue, Moral Distress, and Work Engagement in Surgical Intensive Care Unit Trauma Nurses: A Pilot Study." *Dimensions of Critical Care Nursing* 33, no. 4 (2014): 215–25.

PAGE 223: **In contrast, only a minority:** Mildred Z. Solomon, Deborah E. Sellers, Karen S. Heller, et al., "New and Lingering Controversies in Pediatric End-of-Life Care," *Pediatrics* 116, no. 4 (2005): 872–83.

PAGE 224: **often it is the patient or family members who turn a deaf ear, even if we try:** Zier et al., "Surrogate Decision Makers' Interpretation of Prognostic Information: a Mixed-Methods Study."

PAGE 229: **A recent study in *JAMA Oncology* showed that even active patients with metastatic cancer were apt to have a significant worsening of quality of life from chemotherapy:** Holly G. Prigerson, Yuhua Bao, Manish A. Shah, et al., "Chemotherapy Use, Performance Status, and Quality of Life at the End of Life," *JAMA Oncology* 1, no. 6 (2015): 778–84.

CHAPTER EIGHT: SHARING THE JOURNEY

PAGE 233: **In June 2014** *The New York Times Magazine* **published an essay:** http://www.nytimes.com/interactive/2014/06/22/nyregion/rookie-new -york-firefighter-faces-first-test.html?_r=0.

PAGE 245: **A** *time trial*, **or time-limited therapy, is a concept that has been discussed intermittently in the ICU and palliative care literature for a few decades:** David K. P. Lee, Andrew J. Swinburne, Anthony J. Fedullo, and Gary W. Wahl, "Withdrawing Care: Experience in a Medical Intensive Care Unit," *Journal of the American Medical Association* 271, no. 17 (1994): 1358–61.

PAGE 246: **time trials were offered only 15 percent of the time, and even in those cases, they were infrequently and incompletely discussed:** Yael Schenker, Greer A. Tiver, Seo Yeon Hong, and Douglas B. White, "Discussion of Treatment Trials in Intensive Care," *Journal of Critical Care* 28, no. 5 (2013): 862–69.

PAGE 263: **at the Penn State College of Medicine; nearly half of them depict their attending physicians as abusive monsters:** Daniel R. George and Michael J. Green, "Lessons Learned from Comics Produced by Medical Students: Art of Darkness," *Journal of the American Medical Association* 314, no. 22 (2015): 2345–46.

PAGE 263: **medical trainees suffer staggering rates of depression:** Thomas L. Schwenk, "Resident Depression: The Tip of a Graduate Medical Education Iceberg," *Journal of the American Medical Association* 314, no. 22 (2015): 2357–58.

PAGE 263: **In a recent study, 673 students from thirty-one medical schools across the nation were asked to identify aspects of themselves that they felt uncomfortable revealing in their training:** Michael W. Rabow, Carrie N. Evans, and Rachel N. Remen, "Repression of Personal Values and Qualities in Medical Education," *Family Medicine* 45, no. 1 (2013): 13–18.

PAGE 264: **"The pressure to suppress core personal values and qualities may help explain the frequently reported growth in cynicism, depression, and stunted moral growth observed as medical students progress through their training":** Rabow et al., "Repression of Personal Values and Qualities in Medical Education," 17–18.

PAGE 264: **Programs such as The Healer's Art:** David Bornstein, "Medicine's Search for Meaning," *The New York Times Opinionator,* September 18, 2013, available at opinionator.blogs.nytimes.com/2013/09/18/medicines-search-for-meaning.

APPENDIX ONE: A WAY FORWARD

PAGE 290: **Dr. Joanne Lynn and co-workers laid out four typical patterns of functional decline before death:** June R. Lunney, Joanne Lynn, and Christopher Hogan, "Profiles of Older Medicare Decedents," *Journal of the American Geriatrics Society* 50, no. 6 (2002): 1108–12.

PAGE 294: **the work of Ezekiel Emanuel to create the following basic checklist to get you started:** Ezekiel Emanuel. *The Ends of Human Life* (Boston: Harvard University Press, 1991).

APPENDIX TWO: AVOIDING UNNECESSARY SUFFERING

PAGE 299: **Unfortunately, statistics show that increasing numbers of people are dying in pain, according to their surrogates: 61 percent in 2014, a 12 percent leap from 1998:** Singer, "Symptom Trends in the Last Year of Life from 1998 to 2010," *Annals of Internal Medicine,* 175.

PAGE 301: **However, several recent studies indicate that these patients should not receive chemotherapy at all:** Prigerson, "Chemotherapy Use, Performance Status, and Quality of Life at the End of Life," 778. Kneuertz et al., "Overtreatment of Young Adults with Colon Cancer," 402.

PAGE 301: **"If an oncologist suspects the death of a patient in the next 6 months, the default should be no active treatment":** Charles D. Blanke and Erik K. Fromme, "Chemotherapy Near the End of Life First—and Third and Fourth (Line)—Do No Harm," *JAMA Oncology* 1, no. 6 (2015): 785–86.

PAGE 302: **Increasing numbers of patients are receiving implantable cardioverter defibrillators:** Harry G. Mond and Alessandro Proclemer, "The 11th World Survey of Cardiac Pacing and Implantable Cardioverter-Defibrillators: Calendar Year 2009—A World Society of Arrhythmia's Project," *Pacing and Clinical Electrophysiology* 34, no. 8 (2011): 1013–27.

PAGE 302: **while almost all doctors surveyed agree that deactivation is appropriate in terminally ill patients, these conversations happen only 27 percent of the time:** Nathan E. Goldstein, Rachel Lampert, Elizabeth Bradley, et al., "Management of Implantable Cardioverter Defibrillators in End-of-Life Care," *Annals of Internal Medicine* 141, no. 11 (2004): 835–38.

PAGE 302: **And even for patients with ICDs who are DNR, for whom death is already expected imminently, the conversations are happening less than 50 percent of the time:** Nathan E. Goldstein, Rachel Lampert, Elizabeth Bradley, et al., "Management of Implantable Cardioverter Defibrillators in End-of-Life Care," *Annals of Internal Medicine* 141, no. 11 (2004): 835–38.

PAGE 303: **Many, including the American Geriatrics Society, advocate that patients with end-stage dementia receive careful hand-feeding instead of using a feeding tube:** Clinical, Practice, and Models of Care Committee, "American Geriatrics Society Feeding Tubes in Advanced Dementia Position Statement," *Journal of the American Geriatrics Society* 62, no. 8 (2014): 1590.

PAGE 307: **In the fifteen years between 1997 and 2012, a total of 673 patients chose to exercise this right:** Health Research Funding, "25 Surprising Physician Assisted Suicide Statistics," July 13, 2014, available at healthresearchfunding.org/physician-assisted-suicide-statistics.

Acknowledgments

It took a village.

This book would never have materialized without the brilliant and loving support of my husband, Mark Zitter. His extensive content and literary input are dwarfed by his relentless encouragement and belief in me and my message.

Marisa Handler, thank you for being a spectacular writing coach and friend. Your profound instinct for telling a story and your calm presence at moments when I could otherwise have gotten derailed were critical to the successful completion of this book.

Thank you to my agent, Jim Levine, who believed in this book right from the beginning and found me the perfect publisher at Penguin Random House. And to the people at Penguin, who believed in my message and put their faith in me, a first-time author, to pull it off.

To Caroline Sutton, my editor at Penguin, who "got it" on so many fundamental levels, thank you for providing excellent guidance and counsel.

I would like to thank Pat Murphy, Dr. Anne Mosenthal, and the Family Support Team (now the Palliative Care Team) at University Hospital in Newark, New Jersey, who demanded that I practice patient-centered medicine, even before I could hear them, and then took me under their collective wing to teach me how to do it.

Thank you to my many friends, family members, and colleagues, particularly Yoav Rekem, Sarai and Sherry Zitter, Rhoda Nutik, Felice Maranz, Denise Rekem, Jane Wolk, Monica Bhargava, Angelo Volandes, Dara Lee, and Laura Mazer, who read my book before it was readable and commented tirelessly and honestly in ways that energized and encouraged me.

To my parents, Drs. Rhoda and Stephen Nutik, thank you for believing in me from the start and inspiring me to be my best self.

To those family members who shared details about the lives of my ancestors—Allen Nutik, Lynne Besen, Sandra and Norman Samuels, Wes Golomb, Audrey Browne, and Dora Ullian—thank you for helping me bring richness to their stories.

To my children, Solomon, Tessa, and Sasha, thank you for forgiving my frequent absences and distractions while I wrote this book and for loving me all the same.

Thank you, Dan Krauss, for facing your own fears in order to create *Extremis,* the beautiful, award-winning documentary about these issues, filmed in our ICU.

To my wonderful colleagues on the Highland Hospital Palliative Care service, particularly our social worker Anne James, who took many late-night calls to clarify patient details and enthusiastically encourage this project, thank you. Thanks also to Linda Bulman, Betty Clark, Sheira Freedman, and Claudia Landau, for the constant inspiration and support to do this very difficult work.

To the staff of the Highland Hospital Intensive Care Unit, including my physician colleagues, nurses, and all of the trainees with whom I have worked, thank you for fostering a medical environment that has encouraged me to put my values into practice.

My thanks to Brian Shaw, who did amazing work as my research assistant despite being a third-year medical student and planning a wedding.

I am grateful for the wise counsel of my beloved rabbi, Judah Dardik, who checked and rechecked all of my discourse on Jewish history and law.

Thank you to my Northern California Palliative Care support group, including Shoshana Ungerleider, Dawn Gross, Ken Rosenfeld, Katy Butler, Louise Aronson, Meredith Heller, Sherry Goldyn, Melissa Stern, and others, who bring laughter and Bay Area creativity to the solemn work that needs to be done.

My heartfelt gratitude to all of the health care providers, past, current, and future, working to reshape the existing paradigm of medical care, both within the ICU and outside of it, trying to redirect our efforts toward the well-being, not just the being, of the patient.

And last, I would like to thank my patients, most of whom are no longer with us. You have taught me in so many ways about the importance of listening to the patient and trying to be the most compassionate and caring person I can. I hope that I have made your lives a little bit better, and if I didn't, I ask your forgiveness. What you taught me will be put to good use.

Index

Advance Care Planning Decisions, 270

Advance Directives, 78–80, 134, 150, 190, 198–99, 204–7, 221, 289, 296, 297, 310

Advanced practice registered nurses (APRNs), 22

Africa, 156

African Americans, 68, 149–53

Agitation, 49, 117, 178, 220

AIDS, 46, 225–26, 254

Alexander, Larry, 25

Altilio, Terry, 236

Alzheimer's Association, 292

American Academy of Hospice and Palliative Medicine (AAHPM), 151, 236

American Board of Internal Medicine, 55, 71

American Board of Medical Specialties, 45

American Medical Association Code of Medical Ethics, 66–67

American Society of Clinical Oncology, 139, 306

Anna Karenina (Tolstoy), 186

Annals of Internal Medicine, 131

Antibiotics, 40, 48, 73, 87, 213, 242–43, 295, 297
  bacteria resistant to, 135
  for pneumonia, 58, 176, 244

Anti-HIV medications, 225

Anti-Semitism, 6, 8

Anxiety, 167, 178, 186, 226, 258–59, 268
  of family members, 166, 175, 207
  of health care providers, 222

Aortic aneurism, 11

Ariadne Labs, 311

Arm restraints, 82–83, 117, 124, 176

Arrhythmia, 35–36, 79, 93, 243, 302

Asthma, 4

Atropine, 5

Auschwitz, 57

Autonomy, 66, 68–71, 154–55, 257, 259, 294, 303

    excessive adherence to honoring, 90, 92, 133–36, 145, 150

Barry (heart disease patient), 131–33, 137, 223, 269

Bedsores, *see* Pressure ulcers

Being Mortal (Gawande), 143

Berkowitz, Baruch, 252

Big Three, 85, 86, 94

Bioethics, 41, 50, 69, 86, 137, 170

Biopsies, 109, 143, 164, 182, 195, 197

BiPAP oxygen masks, 59–61, 88–89, 224–25

Bisphosphonates, 201, 202

Blank, Helen, 50–54, 69

Blanke, Charles, 301

Bleeding, 20, 84, 176, 213, 299–300

    in brain, 85, 86, 111–13, 127

    gastrointestinal, 74, 87–88, 92, 94, 239

Block, Susan, 143

Blood clots, 44, 105, 111–13, 124, 239, 267, 268

Blood pressure, 20, 26, 107, 162, 175, 227, 256

    high, 82, 111, 124

    low, 20, 49, 87, 88, 107, 126, 175, 188, 281

    support medications for, 48–49, 74, 87–88, 108, 117, 124, 133, 157, 182, 238–39, 242, 243, 273

Blood transfusions, 10, 84, 93, 94

Book of Life, 277

Bowel obstructions, 57, 196, 197, 248, 300

Brain, bleeding in, 85, 86, 111–13, 127

Brain lesions, 14

Breast cancer, 19, 69, 100, 201, 256, 258

Breathing machines, *see* Ventilators

Brigham and Women's Hospital (Boston), 17–18, 30, 72, 143, 251–53

Bronx County Medical Society, 132

Brown University, 274

Buddhists, 98, 275

Buttonwood Court independent living facility, 198–200

Byock, Ira, 43

California, surrogate legitimacy in, 154

Canadian Army, 10

Cancer Treatment Center of America, 70

Cancer, 44, 66, 123–24, 201, 299–300

    medical treatment of, 72–73, 219, 249–50, 304 (*see also* Chemotherapy; Radiation treatment)

    palliative care and hospice services for, 50, 73, 306–7

    See also Metastatic cancer

Cardiology/cardiologists, 32, 34, 67, 74, 237–38, 251–53

    interventions by, 34, 75, 79–80, 85, 132–34 (*see also* Cardiopulmonary resuscitation)

Cardiopulmonary resuscitation, 2, 4, 26, 31–32, 62, 84, 188
  duration of attempts at, 5–6, 91
  orders prohibiting, 183, 198–99, 296–97, 310 (see also Do Not Resuscitate [DNR] orders)
  patients' decisions not to undergo, 206, 239
  See also Chest compressions; Electric shocks
Carla (ovarian cancer patient), 109–10
Carter, Fred, 187–92
Casarett, David, 106
Case Western Reserve University School of Medicine, 10, 34
Catheters, 2, 31, 33, 62, 72, 79, 83
  dialysis, 19–21, 24–25, 65, 160, 174, 178–80, 206, 213, 303
  Foley, 1
  rapid infusion, 281
  Swan-Ganz, 34–37, 39, 252
Catholics, 77
Center to Advance Palliative Care, 311
Charles (morbid obesity patient), 87–94
Chemotherapy, 62, 138–41, 171–72, 270, 213
  conversations with patients about, 217, 228–30, 258, 282–86
  for metastatic cancer, 19, 100–2, 195–98, 229, 280–81
  "palliative," 100, 301
  palliative care and hospice alternatives to, 73, 109–11, 229, 256, 286–87, 306–7
  patient refusal of, 195–98, 201

Chest compressions, 2, 5, 18, 85, 86, 90, 91, 157
Chief Medical Officers (CMOs), 51
Chinese culture, 156, 172–73
Cirrhosis, 129
Clara (heart attack patient), 192–95
Clark, Betty, 153
Clotting, 20, 88, 94, 129
Code Blue, 3, 50, 55, 86, 173, 227
Codes, 2, 31, 55, 227, 233, 234, 258
  dying patients subjected to, 84, 93–94
  orders forbidding, 105 (see also Do Not Resuscitate [DNR] order)
  response to announcements of, 3–4
  time requirements before stopping, 91
  See also Code Blue
Colon cancer, 195, 198
Columbia Presbyterian Hospital, 138–39
Comatose patients, 33, 51, 124, 133, 188, 211, 256
Comfort measures, 61, 249, 273, 297
  See also Pain management; Symptom management
Computerized tomography, see CT scans
Connors, Alfred, 35–42, 284
Consent, 20, 40, 47, 68, 82, 84, 115, 179
Constipation, 49, 271
Conversation Project, The, 309–10
Cook, Steven, 244–47
Critical care medicine, see Pulmonary and critical care medicine
CT scans, 14, 87–88, 109, 111, 115, 117, 195, 239, 248, 279

Cultural differences, 68, 145, 157–63, 186
sensitivity to, 153–56, 160, 262

Dachau, 132
Dana-Farber Cancer Institute, 143
Danforth, Dr., 183–84
DC defibrillator, 252, 254
Death Cafes, 169–70, 310
Death over Dinner, 310
"Death panels," 51
Decubitus ulcers, *see* Pressure ulcers
Delirium, 49, 57, 60, 109, 117, 138, 140, 142, 178, 209, 268
Dementia, 152, 188–89, 206, 211, 290
end-stage, 175–78, 208, 220–21, 292–93, 302–3
Depression, 87, 104, 116, 156, 186
among health care providers, 95, 218, 222, 263–64
Designated power of attorney, 205
Deuteronomy, 7
Dialysis, 85, 88, 126, 130, 243–44, 246, 272, 295, 303–5
catheters for, 19–21, 24–25, 65, 160, 174, 206, 213, 278–80, 303
Differential diagnosis, 29
Diminished capacity, 192–95
Don (melanoma patient), 270–74
Do not intubate (DNI) order, 240
Do Not Resuscitate (DNR) order, 79–80, 93, 108, 125, 199, 240, 261, 296, 297
Dreux, Roland, 163–68
Drinker respirator, 25
Duke University, 151
Duty, sense of, 178–80
Dysfunctional families, 183, 186–87, 191–92

Electric shocks, 85, 86, 90, 157, 297
Ellen (palliative care social worker), 104, 105
Emanuel, Ezekiel, 294
Emergency Medicine Technicians (EMTs), 296
Emergency rooms (ERs), 10–11, 57, 75, 139, 176, 178, 188, 195, 225, 296–97
author's childhood experience in, 15–16
intubation in, 81, 111, 117, 163
patients moved to intensive care unit from, 60, 124
symptom management in, 138
Emphysema, 3, 40, 142, 144, 148, 291–92, 299, 306
Epinephrine, 5, 91–92
ER (television show), 86
Ethiopian culture, 172
Euthanasia, 42, 165, 307
Exodus, 7
Extracorporeal Membrane Oxygenation (ECMO), 304–5

Family dysfunction, 183, 186–87, 191–92
Family Support Teams, 22, 45–46
Family of Woman, The (Mason), 9
Feeding tubes, 77, 85–86, 174–77, 198, 243, 295, 300–3
percutaneous endoscopic, 44, 81–82, 184, 207, 269
Fistula, 179
Five Wishes, 310
Fluoroscopy, 34
Foley, Kathleen, 44
Foley catheter, 1

Food, cultural attitudes toward,
171–74
Fromme, Erik, 301

Gangrene, 243
Gastroenterologists, 72–74
Gastrostomy tubes, 197, 248–51, 300
See also Percutaneous endoscopic
gastrostomy(PEG) tubes
Gawande, Atul, 143, 267
Get Palliative Care, 310
Go Wish Card Game, 310
Greece, ancient, 8, 105–6
Green, Marcia, 279–88
Greenfield (vascular) filter, 44

Hains, Samuel, 124–28
Halacha, 170
Hancock, Bobby, 195–98
Harvard University:
Law School, 132, 137
School of Public Health, 25
Healer's Art program, 264–66
Health insurance, 51, 53, 163
Heart disease, 4, 35–36, 79, 93, 152,
242–43, 269, 291–93, 302
Hemodialysis, *see* Dialysis
Hemorrhage, *see* Bleeding
Herbal supplements, 201, 202
Hippocratic oath, 33, 62, 93
Holocaust, 57–58, 68, 109
Homeless patients, 3, 137, 262
Hospice care, 46, 50, 54–55, 73, 220,
256, 298–300, 305–7
chemotherapy and, 100, 110
for dementia patients, 208,
260–61, 285–86
home, 100–101, 140–42, 201–202,
208, 256, 258

racial differences in enrollment in,
150–51
resistance to considering, 220,
229, 230, 260
Humanism, 27–28, 253, 262–66
Hyperventilation, 111

Implantable Cardioverter
Defibrillators (ICDs), 203
India, 156
Infectious disease medicine, 73,
242
Inhalers, 3, 31, 40
Internal medicine, 16, 17, 28, 143,
251
Internet, 70
Intestinal tract:
bleeding in, 74, 87–88, 92, 244,
245, 267
blockage of, *see* Bowel
obstructions
Intubation, 56, 58–59, 82, 83, 91, 117,
143, 152, 178, 193, 214, 225–26,
228, 239, 258
emergency, 83, 117, 178, 226
See also Catheters; Feeding tubes;
Tracheostomy tubes
Iraq War, 271
Iron Cradle, The (Alexander), 25
Iron lungs, 25–26
Italy, 10

Jada (breast cancer patient), 257–261
Jameton, Andrew, 222
Japan, 154–55
Jenny (ICU intern), 261–62
Jeremy (neurological disease patient),
117–23
Jewish General Hospital, 10, 15

Jews, 6–8, 169–60, 172, 277
  Nazi doctors' experiments on, 57,
    68
Johnson, Kimberly, 151
*Journal of the American Medical
    Association (JAMA)*, 36, 99, 263
  Oncology, 131, 229
  Surgery, 198

Kidney failure, 5, 107, 152, 178–80,
    244, 291
  in cancer patients, 19–20, 155–56,
    160, 182, 213, 271–73, 304
  treatment for patients with, *see*
    Dialysis
Kleinfield, N. R., 233
Korean War, 11, 26

Lehigh Valley Hospital and Health
    Network, 43
Levy, Mitchell, 98, 274–76, 284
Lidocaine, 15, 21, 35
Linda (heart disease patient), 75–77
Liver disease, 19, 88, 129, 195, 197–98
Long-term acute care facilities
    (LTACs), 95–98, 113, 117, 124,
    148
Lopez, Alma, 248–51
Lou Gehrig's disease, 306
Lown, Bernard, 251–52
Lown Cardiovascular Group, 251–53
Lown Institute, 253, 311
  RightCare rounds of, 266
Lung cancer, 182, 279–80
Lynn, Joanne, 290, 292

Mabel (heart disease patient), 151–53
Magnetic resonance imaging (MRI),
    14, 188

Maimonides, Moses, vii
Mannitol, 111
Mariam (medicine program
    resident), 64–66
Marijuana, 129, 202
Marine Corps, U.S., 11
MASH units, 11, 26
Mason, Jackie, 7
Massachusetts General Hospital, 43
Mayo Clinic, 70
McGill University, 8
MD Anderson, 139
Mechanical ventilation, *see*
    Ventilators
MedicAlert bracelets, 199, 297
Medical culture, 16, 63, 73, 160,
    236–40, 264, 266
  of ICU, 22, 39–40, 91, 215–20
  paternalistic, 66–69, 71, 75, 145
  technology and, 70, 252–53
Medicare, 80, 143
Meditation, 98, 201, 274–76
Meier, Diane, 101
Memorial Sloan Kettering Cancer
    Center, 44
Mengele, Josef, 57
Metastatic cancer, 62, 139, 157, 187,
    287, 291
  chemotherapy for, 19, 100–1, 195,
    198, 229, 280
  complications of, 96, 182, 238,
    258
  palliative care for, 53, 101, 301–2,
    306
MetroHealth medical center, 38
Mexico, traditional healers in, 201
Miller, Donald, 153
Miller, Reverend, 191
Miller, Walter, 138–42

Mindfulness in the ICU conference, 98, 274–76

Montgomery, Field Marshal Bernard Law, 10

Montreal Neurological Institute, 11

Moral distress, 98, 100, 182–83, 220–24, 236

Morbid obesity, 87

Morphine, 56, 59, 61, 202, 209, 260, 281

Mortality statistic, 80–81

Mosenthal, Anne, 43–45

Mount Sinai Hospital (New York), The, 101, 236

Murphy, Pat, 21–23, 25, 43–47, 49, 50, 52, 144, 284

Murray, Ken, 99

My Directives, 310

Nasogastric tubes, 94, 248–49

National Healthcare Decisions Day (NHDD), 311

National Hospice and Palliative Care Organization, 310

Naturopathic treatments, 201

Nazi doctors, 57, 68

Nebulizers, 40

Neonatal ICUs, 26, 223

Nerve conduction studies, 164

Neurological disorders, 117, 120, 188, 193–94, 244, 306

Neurology/neurologists, 13–14, 126–27, 164–65

  pain management concerns of, 44, 49

Neuromuscular diseases, 100, 164, 306

Neurosurgeons, 49, 85, 111–15

New England Journal of Medicine, 106

New Yorker, The, 267

New York Fire Department, 233–34

New York Times, The, 137

  Magazine, 233

9/11 terrorist attacks, 233

North Africa, 10

Nursing homes, 83, 133–36, 167, 188, 199, 238, 296, 306

  palliative care versus quality of life in, 114, 148, 165

Obesity, morbid, 87, 244

OB-GYN, 28, 265

Olfactory nerve, 14

Oncology/oncologists, 72–73, 100–2, 229, 265, 173, 280

  in hospice and palliative care decision process, 101–2, 109–10, 182–84, 219, 229, 272–73, 301, 306

Open Society Institute, 44

Ophthalmoscope, 14

Opioid drugs, 48, 209, 240

  See also Morphine

Optokinetic nystagmus, 14

Oregon, Physician Aid in Dying law in, 307

Orthodox Judaism, 170

Osler, William, vii

Ovarian cancer, 109, 155, 171, 248

PADDLES checklist, 267–69

Pain management, 38, 67, 240, 243, 268, 297

  for cancer patients, 44, 109, 139, 195, 197, 201–2, 219, 251, 273–74

  lack of, before hospital deaths, 37, 108, 134, 137, 150, 299

palliative care for, 45, 48–50, 55,
    103–4, 140, 165, 168, 236
Pakistan, 64, 66
Palin, Sarah, 51
Palliative care, 38, 43–56, 62, 63, 137,
    155, 156, 168, 215, 218–20, 294,
    298, 301–2, 305–308
  board certification in, 55, 208
  collegial support in, 239–41
  conversations with patients and
    family members about, 119–24,
    143, 156–58, 179–80, 182–86,
    193–94, 216, 245, 257–61, 305,
    306
  disease-focused treatment and,
    58–61, 73, 76–77, 80–82, 101,
    109–10, 239–40, 306
  integration into mainstream
    critical care of, 43–46, 57–63,
    238
  for pain and symptom
    management, 45, 48–50, 55,
    103–4, 109, 139, 140, 165, 168,
    196, 202, 209, 236, 248, 251,
    270–71, 299
  protocols for, 50, 55
  stressors on practitioners of,
    218–20, 231, 236
  See also Hospice care
"Palliative" chemotherapy, 100, 301
Pancreatic cancer, 138–39
Paralysis, 111–14, 125, 188, 206
Parkinson's disease, 100
Paternalism, medical, 66–69, 71, 75,
    145
Patient-centered care, xiii, 61–62,
    186, 212, 224, 263, 265, 311
  decision making in, 51, 219
Penn State College of Medicine, 263

Percutaneous endoscopic
    gastronomy (PEG) tubes, 44,
    81–82, 184, 207, 269
Periyakoil, V. J., 99
Persistent vegetative state, 77
Personality disorders, 183, 186
Pew Research Center, 150–51
Physician Aid in Dying (PAD) laws,
    307
Physician Order for Life-Sustaining
    Treatment (POLST), 183,
    198–99, 296–97, 310
PleurX tube, 280
Pneumocystis pneumonia, 225
Pneumonia, 40, 56–58, 77, 178, 200,
    225, 244, 299
  aspiration induced, 96, 135, 176,
    208, 303
  treatment of, 40, 56, 58, 176
Pneumothorax, 20
Polio epidemic, 25–26
Power of attorney, 205
Prepare, 309
Pressure ulcers, 87, 96, 223, 240
Prophylactic treatments, 267, 269,
    287
Progressive neuromuscular disorders,
    164, 306
Project on Death in America, 44
Promoting Excellence in End-of-
    Life Care, 42–43
Promoting Palliative Care
    Excellence in Intensive Care, 43
Prostate cancer, 123, 187, 238
Protocols, 10, 22, 44, 31, 73, 139,
    235, 242–43
  code, 2, 55, 234
  ICU, 48–50, 83–84
Public Health Service, U.S., 68

Pulmonary arrest, 199, 234, 296
Pulmonary and critical care
    medicine, 16, 25, 30, 34–36,
    142, 240
Pulse oximeters, 209

Quadriplegia, 188
Quality of life, 62, 114, 115, 128,
    205–6, 303, 305
  hospice and palliative care
    improvement of, 54, 168–69,
    286, 299, 307
  medical interventions worsening,
    72, 96, 100, 229, 244, 249, 295,
    301
Quinlan, Karen Ann, 27
Quinton catheter, 20, 180

Radiation treatment, 123, 184,
    201–2, 258, 283, 287
Radiology, 92, 188, 249
Rahim, Mrs. (ovarian cancer
    patient), 155–63
Raj, Dr., 183
Reeve, Christopher, 206
Reflex hammer, 14
Religion, 41, 153, 163–71, 186
Respiratory distress, 56, 81, 82, 244
  See also Shortness of breath
Resuscitation, see Cardiopulmonary
    resuscitation
Right to die legislation, 307–8
Robert Wood Johnson Foundation,
    37, 42, 43, 45, 275
Rockwell, Norman, 67, 71, 75
Rosh Hashanah, 277
Rounds, 2, 45, 93, 125, 177, 236,
    262
  palliative care, 215

RightCare, 266
Schwartz Center, 224, 266–67

Saechin, George, 111–15
Saephan, Mr. (kidney failure
    patient), 178–80
Saini, Vikas, 253
Santos, Veronica, 201–2
Saturday Evening Post, 67, 75
Schiavo, Terri, 187
Schwartz Center Rounds, 224, 266–
    67
Sedation, 33, 40, 49, 58, 120, 167,
    202, 244, 268
Septic shock, 17, 87, 126, 129, 188,
    208, 223, 242
  causes of, 135, 188, 213, 238
  post-surgical, 155
Shambhala Buddhism, 275
Shortness of breath, 165, 209, 225,
    271, 280
  palliative care for, 56, 59, 148,
    258–60, 297, 299
Social obligation, 178–80
Social Security, 187
Society of Critical Care Medicine,
    39
Solomon, Mildred, 223
Soros, George, 44, 45
Stanford University, 99
Stevens-Johnson syndrome, 84
StressCare, 274
Strokes, 79, 113, 164, 192, 204, 207
Subspecialties, 16, 32, 44, 45, 71–72,
    80, 85, 265
  Hippocratic oath and, 62
  in long-term acute care facilities,
    97
  palliative care as, 45, 216, 218

Substitute decision making, *see*
Surrogate decision makers
Sullivan, Jordan, 233–34
SUPPORT study, 37–38, 40, 42,
46–47, 299
Supreme Court of New Jersey, 77
Surgeons/surgery, 6, 10–13, 15–16,
33, 49, 80, 103–5, 119, 209, 219
cancer, 155
oral, 11
radiologic guidance for, 88, 92
trauma, 43, 44
tubes inserted by, 40, 82, 84, 135,
165, 195, 216
Surrogate decision makers, 92–93,
131, 145, 187, 223, 226, 235, 299,
304
designation of, 190, 221, 296, 309
for patients on life support, 31, 74,
77, 165–66, 185, 192–94, 300
Surviving Sepsis Campaign, 274
Swan-Ganz catheter, 34–37, 39, 252
Symptom management, 138, 140,
196, 240, 258, 285, 305
See also specific symptoms
Syria, 10

Talmud, 7, 169
Terry (heart disease patient), 78–80
Thirty-day mortality statistic,
80–81
Thoracic surgery, 11
Time trials, 144–47
Tolstoy, Leo, 186
Torah, 7, 169
Tracheostomy tubes, 40–44, 81–82,
174, 188, 195, 269
in long-term acute care facility
patients, 95–96, 148

spontaneous breathing trials
before moving on to, 117–19
talking to patients and family
members about, 119–22,
125–26, 211
two-week decision point for
placement of, 84, 125, 147–48,
165–67, 188–89, 244–47
Tuskegee University, 68, 150
Two-point discriminator, 14

Unetaneh Tokef (Let Us Cede
Power) prayer, 277
University of California, San
Francisco (UCSF), 30, 36,
55–56, 254, 274
Healer's Art program at, 264
University Hospital (Newark, New
Jersey), 18–25
University of Medicine and
Dentistry of New Jersey
(UMDNJ), 43, 45, 50, 133
University of Washington Schools of
Medicine and Nursing, 43
Urinary tract infections, 48, 83, 96,
135, 200

Values, 50–51, 55, 67, 134, 155, 159–60
of medical culture, 102, 200,
265–66
of patients, 38, 75, 82, 121,
144–45, 195–98, 247, 285
of surrogate decision makers, 144,
167, 194, 221
See also Moral distress
Ventilators (breathing machines), 37,
40, 85–87, 91, 192, 213, 220,
226–27, 243, 267–70, 273, 295,
303

Ventilators (*cont.*)
death of patients on, 31, 38, 83, 96, 104, 143, 191, 225, 306
disconnection of patients from, 41–42, 111, 122, 152, 172, 185–86, 213–14, 216–17, 242
emergency room patients on, 81, 163, 282
Family Support Team opposition to, 22–23
in long-term acute care facilities, 95–97, 113, 117, 121, 125
orders prohibiting, 183, 198, 240
palliative care of respiratory distress without, 56
during surgery, 79–80, 114–15
surrogate decision makers for patients on, 74, 190–95
talking to patients about, 152–53, 157, 188–89, 219, 258–60
time trials for, 245–47
tubes connected with, *see* Tracheostomy tubes
weaning patients from, 40, 147
See also BiPAP oxygen masks

Veterans Administration (VA) hospitals, 213–14
Videoscopic X-rays, 34
Vietnamese culture, 172
Vincent (pneumonia patient), 133–37, 223, 269
Vital Decisions, 51–55, 69, 254
VitalTalk, 266, 311
Volandes, Angelo, 270

Wall Street Journal, 39
White, Doug, 246
Williams, Mr. (AIDS patient), 225–28
World War II, 10, 26, 131–32

X-rays, videoscopic, 34

Yom Kippur, 277
Youngner, Stuart, 41
YouTube, 37

Z, Mrs. (pneumonia patient), 57–61, 109
Zen Hospice Project (ZHP), 254–56